A Historical Foundation of CTE in Football Players

Before the NFL, There was CTE

Bennet Omalu, MD

Printed in the United States
Designed by Bookwrights.com

ISBN PRINT: 978-0-9916353-1-3
ISBN EBOOK: 978-0-9916353-2-0

Dedicated to
Prema, Ashly and Mark, my love, my life, my joy.

Contents

INTRODUCTION

In 2003, Dr. Elliot Pellman, the chairman of the Mild Traumatic Brain Injury Committee [MTBIC] of the National Football League [NFL] published an article titled "Background on the National Football League's research on concussion in professional football" (1). Dr. Pellman is a trained internist and rheumatologist. Before his appointment as chairman of the MTBIC in 1994, he had been an associate team physician and internist since 1987 for the New York Jets, an NFL team. In this 2003 article, Dr. Pellman stated the following: "Although published information existed, most of what I – like other team physicians – knew about concussions was from on-field anecdotes passed on from other team physicians and athletic trainers who had been treating professional football players for many years. During my years of medical school, internal medicine training [including an extra year as chief medical resident], and fellowship, from 1975 to 1986, I had never received a single lecture on concussions. As I learned later, this was typical of physician training for what was then an often underdiagnosed and little understood clinical condition." (1).

Dr. Pellman stated that "During my treatment of Mr. Toon, I quickly realized how few experts and how little prospective, scientific medical information were available regarding concussions. I decided that a novel approach would be necessary to gather information, particularly for a professional sports league..." (1), and this new approach was the formation of the MTBIC. He also stated that "It became apparent to the committee that there was no single accepted definition of concussion and that, if we were to begin asking questions regarding the problem, we would need a single definition that would be used league-wide by the medical staffs of all the teams." (1).

Are these statements scientifically valid or are they founded upon the wrong anecdotal premise and assumptions? Assumptions probably based on the calculated inklings of sophisticated agents representing an even more sophisticated principal, the National Football League [NFL], for the purposes of brand management and brand equity optimization. Is it really possible that in 2003 the sports industry, medical and scientific communities did not yet know about concussions and did not understand the clinimetrics, pathoetiology, pathophysiology or sequelae of blows to the head and/or concussions? When and what could the medical and scientific communities have known and reported in the published literature on the association between blows to the head and Chronic Traumatic Encephalopathy [CTE] in high-impact contact sports? Is there really no historical foundational basis for CTE in sports prior to Dr. Pellman's 2003 report?

Two epoch-making and historically valuable reports on CTE in sports were easily identified and reviewed (2, 3). The first report was written by Martland and published in 1928; it described the "punch drunk" state in boxers (2). The second report, the 1937 paper by Millspaugh, renamed the "punch drunk" state "Dementia Pugilistica" [DP] (3). The references cited in these two reports were reviewed, and those references that focused on CTE and the long term outcomes of concussions and traumatic brain injury in sports were identified. The references of these subsequent cited references were also reviewed, and those addressing CTE and the long term outcomes of concussions and traumatic brain injury in sports were selected and examined. Through this process, articles from the present day as well as those dating back to the 17th century B.C. were discovered. Tens of thousands of published reports and references on the subject of traumatic brain injury in sports were encountered. At the end of this review we found and selected 259 published reports and references that described the progressive and foundational link between concussions in sports and CTE; what and when we knew about the historical link between concussions in sports and CTE. These findings are presented in this book under the following six topics:

1. Definition of CTE
2. Post-traumatic encephalopathy [PTE] versus CTE
3. Emerging neuropathology of CTE

4. Definitions of concussions
5. Historical foundation of CTE
6. Historical reports on the neuropathology of CTE

DEFINITION OF CTE

Mike Webster was a deceased retired NFL player who was regarded as one of the best centers in NFL history (4). In 2005, CTE or Mike Webster's Disease [MWD], was described in the brain of this deceased retired American football player as a unique disease entity with a distinctive neuropathology (5) associated with repetitive blows to the head, subconcussions, and concussions.

CTE occurs as a sequela of all types of brain trauma and may result from a single traumatic episode or repeated traumatic episodes. It can occur in and outside sporting and military activities and in all walks of life, including wives who have been physically battered by their husbands (6) and individuals who have received many karate kicks (7). The most publicized sub-type of CTE is DP in boxers, first described as 'punch drunk' in 1928 by Dr. Harrison Martland, the Chief Medical Examiner of Essex County, Newark, New Jersey (2). Over 70 years later, in 2002, another medical examiner, Dr. Bennet Omalu (4, 5, 8-12), who was an Associate Medical Examiner in Allegheny County, Pittsburgh, Pennsylvania, described CTE in professional football players and in professional wrestlers (10, 12), underscoring the essential role the autopsy continues to play in 21st century medical sciences (10, 11).

CTE is defined as a progressive neurodegenerative syndrome, which can be caused by single, episodic, or repetitive blunt force impacts to the head and transfer of acceleration-deceleration forces to the brain. CTE presents clinically after a prolonged latent period as a composite syndrome of mood disorders and neuropsychiatric and cognitive impairment, with or without sensori-motor impairment. CTE can be diagnosed by microscopic tissue examination supplemented with direct tissue histochemical and immunohistochemical analysis. Direct tissue analysis reveals topographically multifocal or diffuse cortical and subcortical taupathy in the form of neurofibrillary tangles and neuritic/ neuropil threads accompanied by topographical low grade to high grade subcortical white matter rarefaction, isomorphic fibrillary astrogliosis, microglial activation, and perivascular and neuropil histiocytic infiltration. Amyloidopathy, TDP-proteinopathy and other proteinopathies may or may not be present. Amyloidopathy may be present in the form of cortical and subcortical diffuse or neuritic amyloid plaques. CTE usually presents clinically after a prolonged latency period; however, some patients with CTE may not exhibit the classic prolonged latency period before clinical symptoms begin (10). The primary proteinopathy of CTE therefore is taupathy, while other secondary proteinopathies may include amyloidopaty, TDP-proteinopathy and/or other proteinopathies.

Starting in 2002, using post-mortem surrogate forensic interviews and interrogations of next of kin of deceased CTE sufferers, Omalu (4, 5, 8-13) identified a constellation of progressive multi-domain neuro-behavioral, neuro-psychiatric, and neuro-cognitive symptomatology which was common to their emerging cohort [Table 1]. In 1927, Osnato (14) had described a similar constellation of multi-domain symptomatology [Table 2] in sufferers of CTE which they termed Postconcussion Neurosis-Traumatic Encephalitis.

POST-TRAUMATIC ENCEPHA-LOPATHY [PTE] VERSUS CTE

PTE is distinct from CTE. PTE and CTE are both sequelae of traumatic brain injury and can occur together in the same individual (10). PTE is not a neurodegenerative disease, and it is not progressive; CTE is a neurodegenerative disease, and it is progressive. PTE is a clinico-pathologic syndrome induced by focal and/or diffuse, gross and/or microscopic destruction of brain tissue following brain trauma (10, 15). Emerging advances in histochemical and immunohistochemical tissue technology enabled a breakthrough case report in 1996 by Geddes et al (16) which reported a case of CTE in a 23 year old boxer using immunohistochemical stains. Geddes' report (16) was substantiated by Omalu's reports in football players in 2005 and 2006 (5, 8), further confirming the distinction between PTE and CTE. In their case report, Geddes et al interestingly noted that the only abnormality detected in the brain of their case was only taupathy without any of the abnormalities previously reported and pathognomonic for DP in boxers (16). Omalu's first case, [Mike Webster] published in 2005, exhibited similar features, but with diffuse amyloid plaques (5). Both cases were typical CTE cases without PTE and showed a topographic distribution of taupathy that was distinct from that of Alzheimer's Disease [AD], relatively sparing the hippocampus (5, 16).

In isolated CTE without PTE, the brain shows evidence of progressive neurodegeneration with proteinopathies [primary taupathy with or without amyloidopathy, TDP-43 proteinopathy or other secondary proteinopathies]. There is no evidence of structural destruction of the brain, and no loss or necrosis of brain tissue. By contrast, in isolated PTE without CTE, the brain shows evidence of structural destruction of the brain with loss or necrosis of brain tissue without evidence of neurodegeneration or progressive proteinopathy.

PTE includes persistent sequelae of primary and secondary brain trauma, including, but not limited to, contusions of the brain, lacerations of the brain, secondary ischemic-hypoxic injury of the brain following brain trauma, ischemic-hypoxic hippocampal sclerosis, intracranial hemorrhages, and compression of the brain, and traumatic cerebral herniations. PTE injuries typically induce necrosis of brain tissue, cavitation and loss of brain tissue, anisomorphic astrogliosis, activation of microglia, and infiltration by histiocytes [either foamy or pigment-laden histiocytes], resulting in scarring of the brain (17-21). A widely recognized subtype of PTE is post-traumatic epilepsy (21-26). Post-traumatic epilepsy originates from a variety of pathogenetic mechanisms, including epileptogenic astroglial scars of the brain and mesial temporal lobe sclerosis (27, 28). When post-traumatic changes similar to PTE occur in the spinal cord a similar syndrome, called Post-Traumatic Myelopathy [PTM], applies. PTE changes are more likely to present with focal lateralizing neurological symptoms and signs (29). They are also more likely to be topographically focal and lobar in the brain (30) and focal and segmental in the spinal cord with attendant Wallerian degeneration of nerve fibers (29).

In the classic CTE cases reported by Omalu (5, 8-13) and Geddes (16) there were no PTE changes. However, CTE can occur with PTE, whereby changes of PTE are present, accompanied by the neurodegenerative proteinopathies of CTE (10). Case #14 of Omalu's reported cohort is a good example of this co-occurrence/ co-morbidity of CTE and PTE (10). This 50 year old professional boxer had suffered a remote severe traumatic brain injury that included a large right acute subdural hemorrhage with cerebral hemispheric compression and cerebral herniation. In addition to CTE changes, his brain exhibited diffuse right cerebral hemispheric multicystic necrosis and xanthochromia [PTE].

To further confirm the distinction between PTE and CTE, Thom et al (31), in their post-mortem series of chronic epilepsy and traumatic brain injury patients, did not find any clear relationship between hippocampal sclerosis, seizure type, seizure frequency, age of onset or duration of epilepsy with Braak staging of taupathy. They did, however, find traumatic brain injury to be associated with taupathy in their series.

EMERGING NEUROPATHOLOGY OF CTE

CTE is not AD but exhibits an AD-like neuropathology. CTE is also not Parkinson's Disease [PD] and does not exhibit PD neuropathology. In younger CTE patients who are more likely to be less than 50 years old, CTE neuropathology is clearly distinct from that of AD; however, as CTE patients get older, the neuropathology of CTE progresses with increasing simulation of AD neuropathology. As CTE advances with increasing age of the patient to end-stage CTE, the neuropathology progressively resembles AD neuropathology (32-37) and may become increasingly more difficult to be delineated from AD in terms of neuropathology (10). In its advanced stages, in older patients who are more likely to be older than 65 years old, end-stage CTE neuropathology resembles AD neuropathology. In its end stages, therefore, CTE neuropathology may be difficult to be distinguished from AD neuropathology. In older CTE patients above 65 years old, the compounding effects of AD, mild cognitive impairment, and normal aging changes in the brain, not related to CTE, may not be reasonably delineated. In older patients above the age of 65 years old who may be suspected to be suffering from CTE, if their brains reveal AD neuropathology without any reasonable distinction from CTE, a diagnosis of AD should be made with a comment that end-stage CTE may resemble AD and cannot be ruled out. Caution should, therefore, be exercised when diagnosing CTE in older patients when AD cannot be ruled out (10).

When PTE and CTE changes co-occur in the brain of the same patient, both PTE and CTE should be reported as co-morbidities. PTE frequently co-occurs with CTE in boxers, who may show evidence of tissue destruction of the brain, including, but not limited to, fenestrations of the septum pellucidum, lobar contusional necrosis, topographic lobar infarcts, and chronic intracranial hemorrhages especially subdural hemorrhages (10, 38-40).

Table 3A enumerates the gross and microscopic changes which may be seen in the brains of CTE sufferers. Table 3B enumerates the four histomorphologic subtypes of CTE which have been introduced by Omalu (10) as the Omalu-Bailes Histomorphologic Subtypes of CTE to facilitate easier identification and diagnosis of CTE based on topographic distribution of neurofibrillary tangles, neuropil threads, and amyloid plaques. CTE sufferers who are also suffering from PTE may show additional PTE changes superimposed on the CTE changes enumerated in Table 3. Similarly, more or different changes may be seen in atypical CTE cases, changes which may deviate from those enumerated in Table 3.

Historically, DP, or punch drunk, has been regarded as a parkinsonian syndrome with motor disorders (39, 40). However with advancing tissue technology, we now know that CTE is not a parkinsonian syndrome and does not exhibit the pathognomonic neuropathology of PD (10), i.e. alpha-synucleinopathy which includes Lewy bodies and Lewy neurites in the substantia nigra and other brainstem nuclei. Rather, CTE is a primary taupathy characterized by neurofibrillary tangles and neuropil threads destroying the substantia nigra and other brainstem nuclei. Though motor symptoms are not the fundamental presenting features of CTE (41-45), if and when motor symptoms occur, they may be driven, in part, by a taupathy or other secondary proteinopathy (46), and not an alpha-synucleinopathy like we have in PD.

CTE has also been historically considered a primary amyloidopathy (16, 21, 47-50); however, immunohistochemistry has demonstrated that CTE is rather a primary taupathy accompanied by other possible secondary proteinopathies, including amyloidopathy (10, 39, 51). Other additional secondary proteinopathies, which may be found in CTE may include, but are not limited to TDP-43 proteinopathy and ubiquinopathy. Mckee (46) has concluded that the presence of TDP-43 proteinopathy in CTE cases meant that motor neuron disease [primary TDP-43 proteinopathy] may be part of the spectrum of CTE, or caused by repetitive traumatic brain injury. This conclusion may be precipitate or premature (52, 53), since TDP-43 proteinopathy may occur as a secondary proteinopathy in a variety of neurodegenerative diseases including AD (54-58).

CTE changes may also be seen in the spinal medulla and anterior horn neurons as part of the long term consequences of repetitive blunt force traumas, and acceleration-deceleration injuries of the head, neck and trunk, and in such instances, the involvement of the spinal medulla does not create a novel disease that is distinct from CTE. The term Chronic Traumatic Encephalo-Myelopathy [CTEM] may be used for such instances, however CTEM is the same disease entity as CTE (46, 59) but with the involvement of both the brain and spinal cord.

Post Traumatic Stress Disorder [PTSD] in military veterans may belong to the CTE spectrum (13). Omalu identified CTE changes in the brain of a 61 year old deceased Vietnam war veteran followed by similar CTE changes in the brain of a 27 year old deceased Iraqi war veteran, both of whom were diagnosed with PTSD (13, 60). The underlying patho-etiology would be similar to that of sports-related repetitive acceleration-deceleration injuries of the brain due to combat and noncombat military activities especially blast exposures, including mortar shells, rocket-propelled grenades, and improvised explosive devices [IEDs] (13, 61-63). Similar to sports-related CTE, other independent researchers (63) quickly confirmed and validated Omalu's findings of CTE-related neuropathology in war veterans diagnosed with PTSD. The link between CTE and PTSD in war veterans remains to be further investigated and may result in the eventual reclassification and sub-classification of PTSD in war veterans as a subtype of CTE [Blast Variant] caused by traumatic brain damage and not simply a neuropsychiatric disease without micro-structural or cellular traumatic brain damage (13). This will delineate PTSD in war veterans from PTSD sufferers who were exposed to strictly emotional and psychologic experiences without physical traumatic brain injury involving transfer of forces to the brain (13, 63).

Omalu (10, 13) has suggested that the clinical symptomatology of CTE as a progressive disease initially involves qualitative impairment of neuronal and axono-dendritic functioning by hyperphosphorylated tau and other possible secondary proteinopathies accompanied by neuropil inflammatory changes, myelinopathy, and astrogliosis. Such impaired functioning results, in part, to an impairment of the delicate homeostatic neurotransmitter milieu of the brain. As CTE progresses with time, there is an accompanying loss of cortical, subcortical and brainstem neurons and axons, which further progresses to expanding impairment with global quantitative deficiency of neurotransmitters in the brain. Multidomain destruction of, and loss of neurons in subcortical and brainstem nuclei will result in quantitative deficiency of a variety of neurotransmitters and neurochemicals synthesized by these damaged nuclei. For example, damage by hyperphosphorylated tau, and death of neurons in the substantia nigra, locus ceruleus, dorsal raphe nucleus and basal nucleus of Meynert will eventually result in quantitative deficiencies of dopamine, noradrenaline, serotonin and acetyl choline respectively, further impairing the homeostatic balance of neurotransmitters in the brain.

While the specific pathophysiological cascades linking traumatic brain injury to CTE have not been clearly elucidated, it is believed that single and repetitive traumatic brain injuries induce upregulation, accumulation, and abnormal enzymatic cellular processing of transmembrane and cytoskeletal neuroaxonal proteins, including amyloid precursor protein and microtubule associated proteins accompanied by cytokine inflammatory and excitotoxic cellular cascades (21, 30, 47, 51, 64, 65) as well as possible seeding, aggregation, and self-perpetuating transcellular propagation [prionopathy] of abnormal pathogenic proteins like hyperphosphorylated tau protein (66-69).

In terms of injury outcomes and risk of CTE, there is emerging evidence that young children and adolescents may possess a higher risk of developing CTE following single and repetitive traumatic brain injury than adults (70-74). This increased vulnerability of CTE by children is, in part, underlaid by their developing and myelinating brain, which responds differently to trauma than the developed adult brain (75-77), and the CTE risk may even be higher the younger the child is (78-80).

DEFINITIONS OF CONCUSSIONS

Concussions and subconcussions are brain and spinal cord injuries caused by acceleration-deceleration forces transmitted to the head and spine by direct blunt force impacts and contact or by acceleration-deceleration forces transmitted to the head and spine without direct blunt force impact or contact with the head, face, neck or trunk. Concussions present with immediate or short-term symptomatic neurological functional deficits, which may impair activities of daily living. Subconcussions do not present any immediate or short-term symptomatic neurological deficit, which may impair activities of daily living (81). Routine conventional neuroimaging studies are typically normal, but may show only brain swelling and edema (73, 82, 83).

Lacerations, contusional hemorrhages, and contusional necrosis of the brain and spinal cord are distinct from concussions and subconcussions and commonly do not occur with concussions and subconcussions. The fundamental and primary underlying neuropathology of concussions and subconcussions are neuro-axonal cytoskeletal and membrane injury and shearing with or without vascular injury. Vascular injury may present with shearing of small caliber penetrating parenchymal blood vessels in the brain with perivascular microhemorrhages. Secondary neuromolecular, neurochemical, and neurometabolic cascades may result in cerebral hypofunction and possibly permanent damage (84). Repeated concussions and subconcussions of the brain and spinal cord can result in long-term, permanent and progressive symptomatic neurological deficits [CTE] (41).

In a consensus statement published in 2011, the American College of Sports Medicine defined a concussion as follows: "Concussion or mild traumatic brain injury [MTBI] is a pathophysiological process affecting the brain induced by indirect biomechanical forces. Common features include the following: rapid onset of usually short-lived neurological impairment, which typically resolves spontaneously; acute clinical symptoms that usually reflect a functional disturbance rather than structural injury; a range of clinical symptoms that may or may not involve loss of consciousness [LOC]; routine neuroimaging studies are typically normal" (82).

In a 2010 clinical report, the American Academy of Pediatrics [AAP] (73) adopted the consensus statement on the definition of concussion by the 3rd International Symposium on Concussion in Sports in 2008, in Zurich, Switzerland (83), which had evolved from the 2001 and 2004 definitions of concussions by the 1st and 2nd international symposia on concussion in Vienna, Austria, and in Prague, Czech Republic respectively (85, 86). The AAP defined concussion as "A complex pathophysiological process affecting the brain, induced by traumatic biomechanical forces and includes five major features:

1. Concussion may be caused either by a direct blow to the head, face, or neck or elsewhere on the body with an 'impulsive' force transmitted to the head.

2. Concussion typically results in the rapid onset of short-lived impairment of neurologic function that resolves spontaneously.

3. Concussion may result in neuropathological changes, but the acute clinical symptoms largely reflect a functional disturbance rather than a structural injury.

4. Concussion results in a graded set of clinical symptoms that may or may not involve loss of consciousness [LOC]. Resolution of the clinical and cognitive symptoms typically follows a sequential course; however, it is important to note that in a small percentage of cases, postconcussive symptoms may be prolonged.

5. No abnormality on standard structural neuroimaging studies is seen in concussion."

In 1997, the Quality Standards Subcommittee of the American Academy of Neurology (87) defined concussions as follows:

"Concussion is a trauma-induced alteration in mental status that may or may not involve loss of consciousness. Confusion and amnesia are the hallmarks of concussion. The confusional episode and amnesia may occur immediately after the blow to the head or several minutes later". The subcommittee divided concussions into three grades. Grade one concussion is characterized by transient confusion, no loss of consciousness and concussion symptoms or mental status abnormalities, on examination, resolve in less than 15 minutes. Grade two concussion is similar to grade one concussion, but for grade 2 concussion, the concussion symptoms or mental status abnormalities, on examination, last more than 15 minutes. Grade 3 concussion is characterized by loss of consciousness, either brief [seconds] or prolonged [minutes].

The chairman of the NFL committee on mild traumatic brain injury [CMTBI] admitted in a guest editorial in 2003 (1) that he and other NFL team physicians did not know much about concussions. Fortunately, they dedicated the first several months of meetings, after their commission in 1994, to the definition of concussions; unfortunately, they "quickly decided" to rename concussions and give it "the more academically appropriate term, mild traumatic brain injury, which is more commonly referred to as MTBI" (1). There was no basis provided for this redefinition or for why members of the committee, who admittedly did not know much about concussions, would think that concussions were mild types of traumatic brain injury without permanent sequelae.

The NFL CMTBI defined mild traumatic brain injury, "after a great deal of discussion", as a "traumatically induced alteration in brain function that is manifested by [1] alteration of awareness or consciousness, including but not limited to loss of consciousness, 'ding', sensation of being dazed or stunned, sensation of 'wooziness' or 'fogginess', seizure, or amnesic period; and [2] signs and symptoms commonly associated with postconcussion syndrome, including persistent headaches, vertigo, light-headedness, loss of balance, unsteadiness, syncope, near-syncope, cognitive dysfunction, memory disturbance, hearing loss, tinnitus, blurred vision, diplopia, visual loss, personality change, drowsiness, lethargy, fatigue, and inability to perform usual daily activities." (1). Interestingly, no mention was made about the possible long term effects and sequelae of concussions, and no mention was made of the risk of permanent brain damage, pathogenesis or diagnostic criteria for concussions.

In 1974 and 1975, Gronwall (88, 89) described concussions as incidents of loss of consciousness at the instant of head trauma, return to alertness within an hour or two, with a period of amnesia, and complete recovery in a few days without objective sequelae. However they acknowledged the persistence of troublesome symptoms in about 10% of cases in the so called post-concussion syndrome (88), which was not accounted for by their description of concussions. They actually opined that there existed objective evidence of a neurosis or persistent objective neurological deficits caused by concussions, which may return to normalcy after about one month [thirty-five days] with a range of 16 to 88 days (88), and frequently lasted beyond one month, which was inappropriate for the time elapsed since injury. According to them, post-concussion symptoms included inability to carry out normal work, poor concentration, fatigue, irritability, and headache (89). They recommended a mandatory and reasonably safe follow-up clinical assessment of concussed patients with persistent symptoms after four weeks of a concussion (89).

In 1964, Dr. Edward Weiford, the President of the Congress of Neurological Surgeons, appointed a committee to study the nomenclature of head injuries. The committee first met on October 6, 1964, and in their subsequent meetings they invited outside consultants from a variety of specialties for "valuable comments" and "inestimable help" during their protracted deliberations, including Dr. Milton Helpern, a forensic pathologist, and the Chief Medical Examiner of New York City (15, 90, 91). The committee was, in part, financed by a United States Public Health Service Grant [1-R01-06066-01] and administered by the University of Cincinnati (15). The committee finally defined a concussion as "a clinical syndrome characterized by immediate and transient impairment of neural function such as alteration of consciousness, disturbance of vision, equilibrium, etc., due to mechanical forces." (15). This committee did not stop at simply defining concussions, they also recognized and defined other post-traumatic and post-concussion syndromes which were "temporally, and implied causally, related to trauma", and included post-traumatic dementia, post-traumatic delirium, traumatic encephalopathy, post-traumatic syndrome [postconcussion syndrome], punch-drunk syndrome, neuropsychological disorder [acute or chronic brain syndrome], post-traumatic epilepsy, etc. (15).

Post-traumatic dementia was defined as "a form of neuropsychological disorder, post-traumatic, with mental impairment". Post-traumatic delirium was defined as "a form of post-traumatic neuropsychological disorder with disturbed consciousness, agitation, hallucinations, delusions, and/or disorientation". Traumatic encephalopathy was defined as a "disturbance of structure and/or function of nerve cells, glia, or intracranial vessels resulting from injury". Post-traumatic syndrome [postconcussion syndrome] was defined as "a clinical complex characterized by headache, dizziness, neurasthenia, hypersensitivity to stimuli, and diminished concentration". Punch-drunk syndrome was defined as "a form of chronic neuropsychological disorder, presumably due to repeated head trauma, often associated with chronic alcoholism, characterized by emotional and/or mental impairment and/or motor deficit". Neuropsychological disorder [acute or chronic brain syndrome] was defined as a "disturbance of mental function due to trauma, associated with one or more of the following: [1] Psychotic manifestation. [2] Neurotic manifestation. [3] Behavioral manifestation. [4] Psychophysiological manifestation. [5] Mental impairment." Acute neuropsychological disorder [acute brain syndrome] lasted up to several months. Chronic neuropsychological disorder [chronic brain syndrome] persisted for months or indefinitely after a concussion or head injury (15).

In 1964, Ward (92) defined concussions "as the loss of consciousness and associated traumatic amnesia, which occurs as a consequence of head trauma in the absence of visible damage to the brain. The absence of morphological damage does not mean that this is not a serious condition, since death can occur from pure concussion as was first documented by Littré in 1705 (93)".

In a 1941 editorial in Archives of Neurology, Denny-Brown

also opined that concussions were the most transitory types of trauma to the nervous system with reversible effects and without detectable pathology (94, 95). However, in a prior 1940 paper, Symonds (96) concluded that the symptoms of concussions could not be made to conform with any arbitrary limit of time, either taken from recovery of symptoms or the absence of symptoms or sequelae, and that there may be no signs of brain injury even when concussions and the symptoms of concussions were severe and prolonged, although in some cases of severe concussions, there may be evidence of local brain injury (96, 97).

In 1927, Miller (98) recommended that "The term concussion should be used to indicate a group of symptoms which are the result of a temporary inhibition of cortical function, with or without stimulation or inhibition of one or more of the medullary centers, but which are not accompanied by pathologic lesions" (98) of the brain. Miller offered a physiologic perspective of concussions and surmised that "the essentials of concussions were an immediate loss of consciousness, with or without symptoms, suggesting medullary effects, and with a progressive tendency toward recovery". However, he also claimed that a pure concussion, which was a concussion without any gross lesion, can cause immediate death (98).

Trotter (99, 100), in his 1924 paper, described concussions as follows: "I may say at once that I use the term concussion, as I think it should only be used in the strict classical sense, to indicate an essentially transient state due to head injury, which is of instantaneous onset, manifests widespread symptoms of a purely paralytic kind, does not as such comprise any evidence of structural cerebral injury, and is always followed by amnesia for the actual moment of the accident". Later in 1927, Osnato (14) affirmed that this definition was generally accepted at this time, however, following their examination of 100 patients with head trauma, they refuted this definition, stating that concussions comprised injury to the brain, and had a potential of causing permanent brain damage or postconcussion neurosis.

In 1874, Koch and Filehne (101) defined concussion as follows: "Concussion is a state of more or less disturbed consciousness with lost or practically lost reflexivity. The appearance is that of sleep or apparent death. There is occasional vomiting. The respiration is slow, shallow and regular, the pulse is weak, slow and generally regular, the pupils are dilated and react sluggishly, the temperature is subnormal" (101, 102).

In 1787, Benjamin Bell (92, 103) distinguished concussions from commotion cerebri when he stated that "Every affection of the head attended with stupefaction, when it appears as the immediate consequence of external violence, and when no mark of injury is discovered, is in general supposed to proceed from commotion or concussion of the brain; by which is meant such a derangement of this organ as obstructs its natural and usual functions, without producing such obvious effects on it, as to render it capable of having its real nature ascertained by dissection." (92).

Barkhoudarian (84) and Giza (104) have enumerated neurometabolic and neuromolecular cellular cascades, which are induced by, and follow a concussion injury of the brain. The cellular events following a concussion may include, but are not limited to, nonspecific depolarization and initiation of action potentials, release of excitatory neurotransmitters, massive efflux of potassium, increased activity of membrane ionic pumps, hyperglycolysis to generate more ATP, lactate accumulation, axolemmal disruption, calcium influx and sequestration in mitochondria, impaired oxidative metabolism, decreased ATP production, calpain activation, initiation of apoptosis, beta amyloid precursor protein overexpression and accumulation, neurofilament compaction via phosphorylation or sidearm cleavage, destabilization of microtubules, axonal swelling, and eventual axotomy.

HISTORICAL FOUNDATION OF CTE

The documented earliest written accounts of the surgical treatment of head injuries in Egypt appeared in the Edwin Smith Papyrus [17th century B.C.] (105), and included 48 cases of trauma; twenty-seven concerned head trauma, six concerned spinal trauma, and principally involved catastrophic head and cervical spinal injuries in military casualties (92, 106). Hippocrates of Cos [born 460 B.C.] (107, 108) noted severe symptoms, including convulsions, following fractures of the skull. Celsus [25 B.C. – 50 A.D.] recognized cerebral hemorrhages following head trauma, without fractures of the skull (108). Hippocrates and Claudius Galenus [2nd centrury A.D.] also described "commotio cerebri" as a broad clinical term that encompassed all injuries of the head, including concussions, cerebral lacerations and intracranial hemorrhages (98). Lanfrancus, in the 13th century A.D., mentioned concussions of the brain when the brain was injured by shaking or severe beating without injury to the scalp or fractures of the skull (108). In the 16th century A.D., Berengarious de Capri [1517] and Ambroise Paré [1575] described concussions as a type of commotio cerebri, which can occur without fractures of the skull (108-111).

With increasing knowledge of brain trauma, especially knowledge of the pathology, the term concussion was progressively limited to injuries of the head, which did not show any clinical evidence or syndrome of increasing cerebral pressure, skull fractures, cerebral contusion or laceration. With the work of researchers like Boirel [1677], Littré [1705], Boyn [1818], Mourier [1834] and Sabatier [on or before 1892] (98, 112), Koch and Filehne [1874], Von Bergmann [1880], Cushing [1908], and others (93, 98, 108-112), the diagnosis of concussion progressively became limited to cases, which did not show any gross lesions in the brain following trauma and culminated in the 1927 paper of

Miller (98), who concluded that concussions were "distinct and separate from contusion or hemorrhages, whether minute or large and diffuse".

Benjamin Bell's definition of concussions in 1787 (92, 103), which has been presented in the preceding chapter, distinguished concussions from commotion cerebri, and his vintage definition withstood the test of time across decades (92). In 1790, Petit (113) also stated in his surgery textbook that commotion cerebri was due to transmissions of vibrations of the skull and blows of the head to the brain, which were more severe without skull fracture (108). However, it was the work of researchers like Boyer [1822], Cooper [1837] and Dupuytren [1839] (114-116) that began to delineate a syndrome of persistent sequelae of commotio cerebri, emphasizing that the effects of concussion may be permanent with somatic and psychic effects (108). Erichsen [1866] (117) was credited with using the term "molecular disarrangement" for the first time when he published a summary of his experiences with railway injuries, and described cerebral and spinal symptoms following blows to the vertebral column without gross injury to the spine, although he was not able to distinguish spinal cord disease from brain disease (108).

In 1889, Oppenheim (108, 118) classified traumatic neurosis, which then was not in general use, to include all neuropsychiatric sequelae of brain injury outside hysteria, neurasthenia and definite organic syndromes which involved underlying functional impairment of the nervous system by mixed organic and psychic factors. Between 1889 and 1921 there was an evolving debate on whether to recognize the cause of post-traumatic clinical brain symptom-complex to be strictly psychic or actual alterations in the brain (108). In 1916, Horn (119) eventually emphasized that there was a distinction between the organic sequelae of injury to the nervous system and the psychologic response to trauma, that the syndrome of "terror neurosis" was distinct from organic post-concussion neurosis. In 1917, Von Sarbó (120) iterated that the so-called functional manifestations of brain trauma were caused by microcellular structural alterations in the brain. Horn's recommendations were later supported by Tromner (121) in 1921 who suggested the term "encephalopathia traumatica" for the organic consequences of injury to the head (108).

Following his examination of 200 brains, Russell (122) reported in 1932 that mechanical agitation of intracranial contents following head trauma resulted in molecular disorganization of myelin sheaths, which formed the organic basis for the persistent symptoms that may follow head trauma. Russell's opinion was similar to those of Erichson (117) and Obersteiner (123) in 1886 and 1879, respectively, both who had proposed molecular disorganization of ganglion cells as the organic basis of persistent symptoms following head trauma (108). Russell (122) also demonstrated widespread astrogliosis in the brain following head trauma, while Stevenson (124) demonstrated microglial activity in the brain following head trauma.

Adolf Meyer, Eugenio Tanzi and Ernesto Lugaro were pioneers in describing persistent and distinctive changes in the brain following neurotrauma. In his 1904 paper, Adolf Meyer (125, 126) presented his findings on the anatomical changes in the brain, and the clinical varieties and symptoms of a syndrome he referred to as "Traumatic Insanity" following brain trauma. He opined that much more severe injuries of the brain accompanied simple cases of concussion than they commonly believed in his time; and concussed patients may present with delayed or persistent insanity even with the absence of major physical damages to the brain. In their book, Malattie Mentali published in 1914 (127), Eugenio Tanzi and Ernesto Lugaro used the terminology "Dementia Traumatica" to refer to persistent symptom-complex and syndrome following brain trauma founded upon localized gross lesions or very mild diffuse lesions in the brain, which were accompanied by a chronic process of gliosis and degeneration of nerves cells. They also described a purely psychogenic syndrome of "Traumatic Neurosis" following brain trauma, which was not founded upon physical lesions in the brain.

During this time, many had believed that concussions of the brain were transient and did not cause any structural damage to the brain especially Trotter (99, 100), who in 1924 defined concussions to include trauma to the brain without any structural cerebral injury followed by amnesia [Trotter's definition of concussion has been presented in the preceding chapter]. A 1923 textbook of legal medicine (128) further stated that nothing definite was found in concussions and inferred that general cerebral congestion, which may accompany concussions, is non-specific and can be found in deaths due to alcohol intoxication.

In 1927, Miller, in his "Cerebral Concussion" paper (98), stated that concussions were not accompanied by pathologic lesions in the brain and can result in immediate death from respiratory paralysis even in cases without pathologic lesions. However, Dr. Miller, in the same paper, opined that concussion was always caused by an impact on the head, which resulted in immediate unconsciousness that was generally accepted as the constant symptom of concussion; most cases were comparatively mild, and there was almost immediate and complete spontaneous recovery. His best example of a mild concussion was "the knock-out blow" in the boxing ring, and stated that it was inconceivable that such knock-out punches in the boxing ring would cause any gross lesions in the brain. Although he admitted that "light blows" on the head often caused transient vertigo, grogginess, "sparks before the eyes" and similar symptoms, he dismissed them to be of little clinical interest since the blows caused only mechanical stimulation of the central nervous system without injuries. He finally concluded that concussions tended to spontaneous recovery without sequelae (98).

However, Osnato and Giliberti, director and associate director, respectively, of the Department of Neurology, New York Post Graduate School and Hospital, challenged this prevailing conception of concussions. In their 1927 paper (14), they stated that concussions were thought to cause no structural damages to the brain because few persons died from simple concussion of the brain and that the number of concussed brains that reached autopsy was so rare that the medical literature was practically barren of concussed brains. Osnato and Giliberti derived the terminology "Postconcussion Neurosis-Traumatic Encephalitis" to describe the sequelae of all types of traumatic brain injuries, especially concussions, based upon their examination of 100 cases of concussion of the brain in a broad variety of traumatic brain injuries. Osnato and Giliberti concluded in this same paper that "...our conception of concussion of the brain must be modified. It is no longer possible to say that 'concussion is an essentially transient state, which does not comprise any evidence of structural cerebral injury'. Not only is there actual cerebral injury in cases of concussion but in a few instances complete resolution does not occur, and there is a strong likelihood that secondary degenerative changes develop...". They further claimed that post-concussion neurosis resembled the neurosis that accompanied encephalitis and should be termed traumatic encephalitis (14). Osnato and Giliberti further identified and enumerated the symptoms and clinimetric prevalences, which they observed in their 100 cases [Table 2].

In a 1939 paper, Schaller recognized the later functional effects of brain injury in patients who had recovered from all acute symptoms of their brain injuries, and entered into a chronic course without gross primary brain injury (102). He recognized this clinical entity by a variety of labels, viz: post-traumatic psychoneurosis, traumatic hysterias, traumatic psychosis, post-traumatic concussion state, traumatic encephalopathy, traumatic encephalitis, cerebral neurasthenia, post-traumatic head syndrome, traumatic constitution, punch drunk state, litigation neurosis, compensation hysteria and concussion neurosis. He opined that these were purely psychogenic states, which developed out of mental complexes following acute symptoms of concussions, which were different from contusions of the brain, that produced temporary inactivity of brain function that may progress to irreversible brain damage (102). Schaller listed the symptoms and signs of the postconcussional state to include headache, vertigo, tinnitus, nervousness, explosiveness, irritability, impairment of memory, impairment of vision, fatigability, poor concentration, sensitiveness to heat and intolerance to alcohol, tremors, vasomotor disturbance and low blood pressure; these symptoms rarely exceeded three months (102). In his opinion, there was sufficient evidence at the time of his paper to delineate the pathologic, clinical and psychic features of this concussion induced syndrome, which was distinct from that of brain laceration and contusion (102). He, however, summarized that the post-traumatic psychoneurotic state was due to psychic complexes in patients with inadequate personality traits and adverse mental influences, opposing the opinion of Oppenheim (129), who had stated that traumatic pyschoneurotic state was due to trauma-induced molecular changes in brain cells (102).

Autopsy and specialized examination of the brains of patients who died in the post-concussion state, long after the initial injury, remained rare (108). In 1929-1930, Haase (130) reported two autopsies of traumatic neurosis, which showed extensive changes in the brain with softening and glial proliferations. According to Strauss in 1934, it was becoming increasingly clear that a psychogenic syndrome could exist following minimal head injury without a clear history of unconsciousness and acknowledged Bennet's (131) 1910 classification of milder forms of concussions of the brain, in which no loss of consciousness occurred at all (108). Strauss (108) opined that concussions were a clinical series of events, which resulted from a blow to the head severe enough to cause a disruption of intracranial equilibrium, and if the blow happened to affect the parts of the brain that maintained the waking state, unconsciousness would result (108). He further opined that significant intracranial injury could occur without loss of consciousness; and failure to fully comprehend or elucidate the pathogenesis of a constellation of emerging psychological symptoms was no proof of psychogenicity or psychoetiology (108). This was in concordance with Russell's assertion that although assessing the presence or absence, and duration of loss of consciousness may be a useful method of evaluating brain injury, it did not always provide an accurate estimate of the degree of cerebral damage (122). Strauss (108) also concluded that negative neurologic examinations and normal mental status should not be the final criteria for determining the presence, absence or degree of damage to the brain resulting from head trauma. He recommended that "traumatic encephalopathy" be used as a generic term to include cases in which post-traumatic physiologic cerebral disturbances were present, but organic brain lesions were not clinically demonstrable (108).

Out of Russell's 141 patients who survived accidental blunt force brain trauma and were examined at a mean interval of six months following injury, eighty-six patients [61%] manifested persistent symptoms of the "post-concussional neurosis or post-concussional syndrome" (122). Physical examination alone was of little value in estimating the degree of cerebral damage, and the chief complaints were headache, dizziness, nervousness, sleeplessness, inability to concentrate, and disturbances of memory and behavior (122).

Critchley (132), in 1949, reported his findings and opinions regarding traumatic encephalopathy in twenty-one punch drunk naval patients. He stated that traumatic encephalopathy was practically and pathologically a progressive and irreversible condition, which advanced steadily even after retirement from a boxing career and cessation of repeated brain trauma. In his cohort, the interval between taking up boxing as a career and development of neurological signs and symptoms of traumatic encephalopathy ranged from 6 to 40 years with a mean of 16 years (132). In a later paper in 1957, Critchley (133) further stated that CTE was based upon multiple minor cerebral contusions, possibly with initial pinpoint hemorrhages later replaced by gliosis, cortical atrophy, and internal hydrocephalus.

In 1957, Graham and Ule (134) contributed their part in the evolving syntax of progressive neurological symptoms in retired boxers when they reported the neuropathological findings in a 48 year old ex-boxer who had developed euphoria, dementia and extrapyramidal impairment. His brain at autopsy showed cortical atrophy and neurofibrillary tangles without amyloid plaques. They suggested that DP be reserved for the chronic progressive disorder, which developed in boxers after a symptom-free latent interval, while the terminology "traumatic encephalopathy of boxers" be reserved for the brain disorders, which occurred immediately following a boxing contest (134).

As medical science and technology evolved, it gradually became even more recognized and established that concussions and repeated blows to the head result in cumulative damage to the brain, and in part, culminated in an epoch-making editorial in the Lancet journal in 1976 (135). This editorial reaffirmed that irretrievable brain damage can occur by many ways including by accident or through disease, and it would rather seem to be a pity to add to the incidence and prevalence of brain damage on purpose through collision sports. Unfortunately, the editorial (135), while incriminating boxing as an avoidable cause of a punch-drunk state, did not apportion similar blame to other contact sports like rugby, soccer, wrestling, horse-riding and football. While recognizing that there may be a risk of brain damage in these sports, the editorial did not recognize that contact sports outside boxing could result in any permanent sequelae resembling a punch-drunk state or traumatic encephalopathy. It recognized repeated minor head injuries and concussions in football and rugby, known as the 'ding', to be short-lived without permanent sequelae (135).

Yarnell and Lynch (136) from the University of California-Davis in 1973, presented the following definition of the ding as described by a professional player: "Getting hit in the head so hard that your memory is affected, although you can still walk around and sometimes even continue playing, you don't feel pain, and the only way other players or the coaches know you've been dinged is when they realize you can't remember the plays". In observing eighteen college football games they had noted an amnestic syndrome in mildly concussed or dinged players comprising a marked transient post-traumatic, impaired short-term memory consolidation with or without brief alteration in consciousness [lasting less than a minute], but with inability to recall an examination within minutes of its completion, a sense of anxious bewilderment and confusion, without marked cognitive difficulty, and only patchy recollection of the episode on recovery, usually within one hour (136). In a previous 1970 paper, Yarnell and Lynch (137) had described four concussed or dinged college football players who manifested post-traumatic retrograde amnesia and confusion. Two of the four players wandered aimlessly about the field after the play had terminated; one stumbled back towards the huddle; another was unconscious for about 30 seconds. The remaining two were initially disoriented to time and place. All four did not know how they left the playing field (137).

The assertion in the Lancet editorial (135) occurred still after Oppenheimer (138) and Corsellis (38) published papers in 1968 and 1973, respectively, confirming that repeated blows to the head, and even a single blow to the head, which could stun a person for a short time, in sporting and non-sporting activities do result in microscopic injuries and changes to nerve fibers, glial and neuronal cells, and penetrating blood vessels of the brain, distinctive patterns of brain damage, nerve fiber and neuronal degeneration, which underlie or contribute to psychological aberrations, impaired memory and dementia, and may not be apparent on naked-eye examination. Oppenheimer went further to state in his summary that these microscopic injuries to the brain were caused by both severe traumatic brain injury and concussions, and could be demonstrated in brain tissues with silver staining techniques within 24 hours of survival after a concussion, and remain visible for many months after the concussion (138). He proposed the following acceleration-deceleration mechanisms of injury: surface shearing and contusion; stretching and tearing of small blood vessels and nerve fibers. He concluded that "The point to be stressed in regard to these cases of 'concussion' is that permanent damage, in the form of microscopic destructive foci, can be inflicted on the brain by what are regarded as trivial head injuries."

Still in response to the Lancet editorial (135), in a letter to the editor in March 1976, Adams (139) stated that there appeared to be reasonable grounds to advise patients to stop collision sports after two episodes of head injury associated with loss of consciousness and/or amnesia. He further opined that in practice unconsciousness may be uncertain, however players who returned to a game after a minor head injury must be observed for delayed-onset of amnesia; and players who sustained cerebral concussion should not be allowed to resume head contact for at least seven days after injury or disappearance of headache, whichever was the longer period.

Fourteen years prior to the Lancet editorial (135), in 1962, Sir Symonds (96), a consulting physician emeritus for nervous diseases at Guy's Hospital, London, had again contested the premise that cerebral concussion was a reversible syndrome without detectable brain damage, and proposed that concussions should include all episodes of unconsciousness whether or not the effects of the injuries were permanent. Sir Symonds questioned whether the effects of concussions, however slight, could be completely reversible. He contended that a patient who suffered from a slight concussion may recover on the short term from the symptoms, but after repeated episodes of concussions there was a gradual appearance of permanent sequelae like in the punch-drunk syndrome in boxers. In such patients concussions may never have been severe, but would have been repeated accompanied by repeated or frequent subconcussive blows to the head, which would result in cumulative concussive injury and brain damage, permanent intellectual impairment and personality disorder. Sir Symonds further surmised that there may be permanent loss of neurons and neuronal function following concussion of any degree, and diffuse loss of neurons may be present after a concussion without any symptoms being apparent either to the patient or an experienced observer. In explaining the latency of permanent brain damage following concussions and the manifestation of functional impairment, Sir Symonds surmised that the number of cerebral neurons is greater than that required for functional efficiency, and in the concussed patient a fraction of the reserve neurons is lost even with complete symptomatic recovery. With repeated concussions, greater numbers of neurons are lost until the reserve of neurons is exhausted and progressive permanent symptoms appear beginning with subjective intellectual problems and subtle personality changes, which may only be observed by a close relative of the patient (96). The same premise of safe cerebral concussion was similarly contested by Ommaya and Gannarelli (95) two years prior to the Lancet editorial.

In a previous editorial in 1961 in the Archives of Neurology, it was stated that the only sign that was unique to cerebral concussion was retrograde amnesia, however Gronwall and Wrightson (88), from the Department of Neurosurgery, Auckland Hospital, New Zealand, were able to demonstrate impaired cognitive functioning in healthy young adults who were twice concussed. They subjected their patients to a simple test of adding serial numbers presented at different speeds. Twice concussed patients processed information at a slower rate than single concussed patients. Recovery was slower in the twice concussed patients although processing ability eventually returned to normal. Partly relying on their data and those of Roberts (40), Gronwall and Wrightson concluded that larger numbers of even mild concussive episodes permanently reduced the speed of information processing, and that repeated blows to the head could result in cumulative damage to the brain. The ages of their study participants ranged from 16 to 26 years old, and the time interval between concussions ranged from 5 months to 8 years (88). They further concluded that: "Whatever the mechanisms for this fall-off in intellectual performance, doctors do have a duty to convince the controlling bodies and participants in sports where concussion is frequent that the effects are cumulative and that the acceptance of concussion injury, though gallant, may be very dangerous."

Unfortunately, sports associations and their doctors pitched concussions as acceptable injuries, and did not accept the premise that repeated concussions and repeated blows to the head in sports can result in sequelae like impaired memory and dementia. When Harvey and Davis (140) reported a case of traumatic encephalopathy in a 25 year old professional boxer in London in 1974, boxing associations and their doctors interpreted it as an excessively rare event in boxing. Even much earlier in 1954, the New York State Boxing Commission had invited Kaplan and Browder and offered them research collaboration in a study on the effects of blows to the head sustained by professional boxers. The boxing commission, Kaplan and Browder (141) reported their study of the brains of professional boxers to confirm that boxing did not cause brain damage. Expectedly they concluded that boxing did not cause the permanent sequelae of punch drunk in boxers. In their study they examined the brains of 1,043 professional boxers in all divisions of boxing using electroencephalography, which was mostly performed within 10 minutes of the cessation of a bout, either at the offices of the New York State Boxing Commission or at the Eastern Parkway Boxing Arena in New York City. They opined that there was no evidence that blows to the head and/or concussions caused permanent brain damage or punch drunk in boxers (141). McCown (142, 143), the medical director of the New York State Athletic Commission proudly reiterated the opinions of Kaplan and Browder in two additional papers he published in 1959 defending the sport of boxing. McCown stated that the punch drunk syndrome or CTE "had never been proven to be a neurological syndrome peculiar to boxers and produced by boxing. It has, unfortunately, become a slick medical cliché with which to label any boxer whose performance and behavior in or out of the ring is unsatisfactory or abnormal". In his summary he concluded that "No clinical or laboratory evidence was found which would substantiate the so-called punch-drunk syndrome that has so often been erroneously identified with boxers" (143). McCown (142, 143) inferred that since the statistics of the New York State Athletic Commission confirmed only seven fatalities over a fourteen year period [1946 – 1951: seven deaths; 1952 – 1958: zero death], boxing was a relatively safe sport as compared to American football and baseball, which showed higher fatalities (144). Paradoxically, McCown recognized that "boxing has often been considered the most dangerous of all the competitive sports" (142).

Still much earlier in 1934 and 1937, Parker (145) and Winsterstein (146) had commented respectively that the cause of punch drunk in boxers was continued "hammering" of the head, and multiple small injuries to the brain affected different systems of the brain at the same time, which was responsible for the varied clinical picture of the punch drunk in boxers; and remissions or recoveries from the punch drunk symptoms may occur if a boxer gave up fighting at an early stage.

It is also rather interesting to note that concussions became the underlying justification and rationalization for the introduction of helmets into American football. According to the NFL encyclopedia (147), the 1888 annual rules convention of college football passed a rule permitting tackling below the waist allowing players to bunch themselves round the runner to protect him rather than arraying themselves across the breadth of the field of play. The emerging game of football became a more savage game necessitating the use of protective gear, pads and helmets. Players did not like wearing these protective clothing; however as time went by more players braved being called sissies to wear them. The helmet was the last gear to be accepted, first the banal head harnesses and then the leather helmets, which were disdained by a macho few. Even the great Glenn [Pop] Warner was known to have counseled his players in Carlisle, Pennsylvania against wearing helmets in 1912 saying: "Playing without helmets gives players more confidence, saves their heads from many hard jolts, and keeps their ears from becoming torn or sore. I do not encourage their use. I have never seen an accident to the head which was serious, but I have many times seen cases when hard bumps on the head so dazed the player receiving them that he lost his memory for a time and had to be removed from the game" (147).

Wearing the helmet was not a mandatory piece of equipment in college football until 1939. The NFL did not require the wearing of helmets until 1943, although most players were already wearing them in games (147). Allegedly, 1940 was the last year a NFL player played in a game without wearing a helmet. George Barclay of Lafayette College has been credited by some with developing the first protective football head gear in 1896. He had it made by a harness maker, and became known as a head harness (147). Three years prior, U.S. Naval Academy midshipman Joseph M. Reeves, who later became an admiral and the pioneer of carrier aviation, had a protective device made for his head out of mole skin to allow him to play in the 1893 Army-Navy Game. He had allegedly been told by a Navy doctor that he must give up football or risk death or insanity if he took another impact to his head from football. Cadet Reeves had gone to an Annapolis shoemaker and asked that a crude leather protective gear be made to protect his head. This later became the basis for the first aviator caps and helmets (148). Contraptions of these head harnesses were developed and eventually evolved into helmets in 1939 when Gerry E. Morgan and other employees at the John T. Riddell Company in Chicago invented and patented a plastic football helmet. These helmets were worn for the first time in a game by some players in the Chicago College All-Star Game of 1939 (147). Ironically, while helmets constitute a vital part of head injury prevention and do reduce the incidence of abrasions, contusions and lacerations of the scalp and face, fractures of the facial skeleton and the skull, intracranial hemorrhages, cerebral contusions and lacerations, they, unfortunately, do not prevent concussions of the brain (73, 149-152).

In his editorial in October 2003 titled "Tackling concussions in sports." (153), the NFL commissioner, Paul Taglibue, touted the NFL's advancing understanding of concussions predicated upon the research and recommendations of the CMTBI, which he appointed in 1994 and saluted in his editorial for their leadership. In this epoch-making editorial, Mr. Taglibue high-lighted safety-related rules changes, advances in equipment development and helmet redesigns by the Riddell Company [manufacturers of NFL helmets] as the league's accomplishments in response to their better understanding of the science of concussions (153). This editorial accompanied the 2003 journal publication of the research findings of the CMTBI, which had planned to embark on a series of research projects aimed at defining the biomechanics of concussion impacts with a major focus on the helmet as the technological tool for the control and management of the epidemic of concussions in football (1, 154).

By the 1990's there was an increasing recognition of the manifesting burdens of repeated concussions on NFL players who were retiring prematurely because of concussion-induced brain damage (155); including players like Al Toon [New York Jets] and Merrill Hoge [Pittsburgh Steelers] in 1992 and 1993, respectively (1). This had been the premise of the creation of the CMTBI, although the membership pre-requisites and qualifications of this committee remain unclarified (1). Surprisingly, the NFL had asked in 1994, when the committee was created, if concussions were a new problem, a misdiagnosed, or an unrecognized problem; whether the sequelae of concussions were statistical anomalies or the beginning of an epidemic? (1, 155). Headed by Dr. Pellman, this committee performed a variety of research projects and published numerous papers to answer the aforementioned questions about concussions (150, 154-169). It is pertinent to note, that right from the onset, the NFL and the CMTBI chose to publish their research findings, analyses and conclusions only in one journal, and pre-selected a single journal to publish all their papers (1). Unfortunately, the committee failed in identifying or recognizing CTE, which was the fundamental objective of their founding; and even denied and dismissed the existence of CTE when it was identified by an unexpected source, Dr. Omalu (5, 8, 170-172). In the opinion of the committee, there was a small number of athletes in whom persistent symptoms of concussions developed [post-concussion syndrome] and precluded them from returning to play for an extended period; and often the post-concussion symptoms were seen one or more weeks after the injury that was usually mild; and consisted of a combination of the symptoms and signs that occurred after a concussion. In the summary of their research findings, no allusion whatsoever was made to CTE or permanent brain damage caused by concussions (155); however repeated allusions were made to post-concussion syndrome in reference to return to play guidelines. The committee stated that "Another often-expressed concern underlying the development of mild TBI guidelines is the occurrence of chronic brain damage as a result of multiple head injuries. A recent letter to the editor in Neurosurgery addressed the case of an NFL player who was alleged to have died of complications of chronic traumatic encephalopathy, underscoring this concern (171). Chronic traumatic encephalopathy in boxers is a well-accepted and documented clinical and pathological syndrome. The clinical features include a combination of cerebellar, extrapyramidal, and pyramidal dysfunction, along with cognitive and personality changes. In the NFL study, none of these features was identified in any player, including those with repeated injury. There were no signs of chronic traumatic encephalopathy in this group of active, contemporary football players" (155, 173, 174).

In yet another epoch-making paper (161), the NFL and the CMTBI claimed that their research showed that it was safe and actually safer and better to return a concussed player to the same game in which he was concussed in spite of generally accepted basic science principles (175). They concluded that "Players who are concussed and return to the same game have fewer initial signs and symptoms than those removed from play. Return to play does not involve a significant risk of a second injury either in the same game or during the season." They further stated: "The results of this article indicate that many NFL players can be safely allowed to return to play on the day of injury after sustaining an MTBI." (161) and actually suggested that their analysis and conclusion in professional football players may have relevance and may be applied to college and high school football players (161). In yet another review paper for neurologists, the NFL and CMTBI concluded and recommended, based on their research, data and analyses, that there was no clinical outcome difference between a single concussion and repeated concussions in a professional football player, and actually reaffirmed that returning a concussed player to the same game reduces the total number of clinical signs and symptoms (173, 174).

In his 2003 guest editorial (1), the chairman of the CMTBI of the NFL, who was a team physician for the New York Jets, stated that he, like other NFL team physicians, did not know much about concussions, although published information existed (1). What the team physicians knew was founded upon on-field anecdotes, which were passed on from other team physicians and athletic trainers, who had been treating professional NFL players for many years. The NFL executives and team physicians only took notice of the possible long term effects of repeated concussions in 1993 after Merrill Hoge retired (1), and Dr. Pellman was summoned to become the chairman of the CMTBI by the NFL commissioner, based on Dr. Pellman's experience with Al Toon, who was allegedly the first professional NFL player noticed to have retired from the NFL because of the so-called post-concussion syndrome. Dr. Pellman had been the team physician of the New York Jets since 1987 and had treated Al Toon. According to Dr. Pellman's editorial, "From the beginning of his professional career, Mr. Toon began to incur what we now recognize as concussions. These 'dings', as they were referred to then, were minor, often causing no more than mild headaches, malaise, intolerance of loud noises, depression, and emotional lability after what were viewed as mild, inconsequential blows to the head. Mr. Toon was experiencing what we now call post-concussion syndrome, which would eventually lead to the premature retirement of this great athlete in 1992. He was the first documented NFL player that I know of to retire as a result of this problem" (1, 154).

Similar to the NFL, Governor Dewey of New York State appointed the very first medical advisory board for the New York State Athletic Commission in 1948 (142, 143). The board consisted of nine members, including a chairman and outstanding specialists and authorities in sports medicine, including a neurologist, psychiatrist, orthopedic surgeon, ophthalmologist, internist, general surgeon, dentist, and a specialist in industrial medicine. These specialists were regarded as experts in fields of medicine that pertained to the medical aspects of boxing, yet it appears that there may not have been a neurosurgeon on the committee despite the prevalence of subdural hemorrhages in boxing (40). The committee was charged with formulation of plans and standards for the medical examination of boxers; recommendation of safety measures, which were necessary for adequate protection of boxers in the ring; recommendation of a panel of physicians for the examination of boxers and wrestlers; preparation of medical forms like the licensing examination forms and accident forms; preparation of a modern medical unit file system; and recommendation of the staffing and equipping of a modern medical office with adequate modern clinical and laboratory equipment. Prior to this time, the local clubs and boxers' managers assumed the financial responsibility for the medical welfare of their boxers. However and unfortunately, the stance of Dr. McCown, the medical director of the New York State Athletic Commission, during this time, was that boxing was a relatively safe sport that rarely, if at all, caused brain damage in boxers (142, 143). Just like the NFL CMTBI, the medical advisory board of the New York State Athletic Commission undertook scientific research, which showed that there was no evidence of permanent brain damage in boxers (141). According to Dr. McCown, the medical advisory board was successful because the fatality rate of boxing in New York State dropped from seven deaths in 1946 to 1951, to zero death in 1952 to 1958 (142, 143) based upon the medical measures and recommendations advocated and adopted by the medical advisory board and the New York State Athletic Commission for the safety and welfare of boxers. He opined that professional boxing will survive and prosper under the measures and programs they had implemented (142).

Still with a focus on fatalities as a measure of safety, Gonzalez (144), the chief medical examiner of New York City from 1935 to 1954 reviewed the causes of death in a variety of sports over a 32 year period from 1918 to 1950. He examined deaths in aquatic competitive sports, body contact sports [American football, wrestling, boxing, hockey and basketball]; sports in which missiles are thrown by hand or with weapons [baseball, cricket, golf, hockey and archery]; and sports in which falls or other miscellaneous accidents may occur [horse racing, polo, handball, basketball, track and field events]. In total there were 104 fatalities in these sports with baseball, American football, and boxing having the largest numbers of fatalities, 43, 22 and 21, respectively, with these three sports representing 83% of all fatalities (144). Based on his data and perspective as a medical examiner, just like Martland (2), Gonzalez asserted that "Thirty-two years of boxing competitions, however, have produced fewer deaths, in proportion to the number of participants, than occur in baseball or football and far fewer deaths than result from daily accidents. It seemed that the moral and physical benefits derived from boxing far outweigh the dangers inherent in it or any of the other competitive sports" (144).

In 1928 when Martland (2) described the punch drunk state in boxers, he asserted that mild to severe forms of the disease occurred in about 50% of boxers especially boxers with long careers, and that there was good evidence to classify the punch drunk state as an occupational disease due to boxing-induced brain injury. Martland believed that boxing induced brain injury was caused by single or repeated blows to the head or jaw, which caused multiple concussion hemorrhages in the deeper portions of the cerebrum, almost never involving the cerebral cortex or below the tentorium cerebelli. The acute premise of the punch drunk state, he propounded, was minute contusional hemorrhages occurring in the brain caused by blows to the head, a proposition, which was based in part on Cassasa's 1924 report (176), which reported the presence of multiple perivascular punctate cerebral hemorrhages in five autopsies of decedents, who suffered and died from head injuries. These five cases showed no lacerations of the scalp, fractures of the skull, major meningeal hemorrhages, cortical lacerations or contusions. According to Cassasa, his cases showed tissue evidence of concussions with isolated multiple perivascular punctate parenchymal hemorrhages without other traumatic lesions of the brain, which he thought to be very rare fatalities, having identified only five cases over ten years at the New York Medical Examiner's office (176). Martland thought that these parenchymal hemorrhages, with time, were replaced by gliosis and progressive degenerative lesions in those who survived such injuries. He interpreted the symptoms in mild and severe forms to resemble those of the so called parkinsonian syndrome (2), including slight unsteadiness in gait and equilibrium, staggering, propulsive gait, slowing of muscular action and movement, marked dragging of one or both legs, hesitancy in speech, tremors of the hands, nodding movements and/or tilting of the head, vertigo, deafness, parkinsonian facies, and slight mental confusion to marked mental deterioration (2). In his paper, Martland stated the following: "I realize that this theory, while alluring, is quite insusceptible of proof at the present time, but I am so convinced from my former studies on post-traumatic encephalitis that this is the logical deduction that I feel it my duty to report this condition" (2). In order to further support the punch drunk state, Martland referred to the previous work of Osnato and Giliberti in 1927 who had concluded, after examining the brains of 100 deceased concussed patients, that concussions can cause permanent brain damage and degenerative brain disease (14). Martland also concluded that in about 2.9% of fatal head injuries, concussions can result in sudden death without any other evidence of brain trauma at autopsy except for multiple perivascular punctate parenchymal cerebral hemorrhages [ring or concussion hemorrhages], possibly accompanied by minimal, focal subarachnoidal hemorrhages. These hemorrhages would be replaced by gliosis and degenerative changes in the brain, which will form the pathophysiologic basis of the post-concussion neuroses and psychoses, following blows or falls on the head, including the punch drunk state in boxers (2). He further stated that this "...condition can no longer be ignored by the medical profession or the public. It is the duty of our profession to establish the existence or non-existence of punch drunk by preparing accurate statistical data as to its incidence, careful neurologic examinations of fighters thought to be punch drunk, and careful histologic examinations of the brains of those who have died with symptoms simulating the parkinsonian syndrome." (2).

In 1937, Lieutenant Millspaugh (3) of the United States Navy Medical Corps was the first to use and propose a new terminology, dementia pugilistica [DP] to describe the punch drunk state in boxers. In his opinion, punch drunk was a colorful but non-distinctive term similar to the other terminologies of concussions of the brain, including post traumatic neurosis or psychosis, traumatic encephalitis and traumatic encephalopathy. To him punch drunk was a derisive connotation; however, DP ruled out related but nevertheless distinct traumatic brain injuries and supplied a distinctive term for a definite condition (3) since mental unbalance encountered in boxers was also observed in athletes in other sports who sustained considerable brain trauma. Millspaugh went further to confirm that DP was a combined physical and psychic syndrome that was caused by head trauma, which was usually repeated and frequent, and varied from comparatively insignificant abrasions, contusions and lacerations, brain concussions and skull fractures to more severe head injuries that could result in traumatic shock, coma, and even death. He concluded that: "Again, repeated and frequent concussions, occasionally very severe, often undoubtedly associated with intracranial capillary hemorrhages, are to say the least not conducive to stabilized mental equilibrium" (3).

Martland's propositions in 1928 about the punch drunk state (2) instigated a contentious debate about the occupational hazards of boxing over ensuing decades culminating in a 1962 debate in the United Kingdom House of Lords (177). The issue of the medical aspects of boxing was referred to the Royal College of Physicians of London by Lord Brain for an independent and scientific investigation by the college to provide facts needed for a more accurate assessment of the dangers of boxing (177). The Committee on Boxing was commissioned and chaired by Lord Brain "to report on the medical aspects of boxing from the data at present available". Lord Brain died in December 1966, before the final report of the committee was published in October 1969. Members of this committee included but were not limited to five neurologists, one cardiologist, one neuropathologist, one ophthalmologist, one thoracic surgeon, one neurosurgeon, and one epidemiologist (177).

The committee sought advice and evidence from a broad variety of associations, specialists and experts in the sporting, medical and surgical fields including the Association of British Neurologists, the Society of British Neurological Surgeons, the Ophthalmological Society of the United Kingdom, the Royal Medico-Psychological Association, the British Cardiac Society, the Society of Thoracic Surgeons, the British Neuropathological Society, the British Association of Urological Surgeons, the Coroner's Society, the Association of Police Surgeons, the Medical Officers of Schools Association, the Medical-Directors-General of the Armed Services, medical officers in charge of professional and amateur boxing, the British Boxing Board of Control, and the Amateur Boxing Association (177).

The committee appointed Dr. A. H. Roberts (40) in 1967 as a research scholar to clinically investigate a random sample of two hundred and twenty-four professional boxers who were registered with the British Boxing Board of Control between 1929 and 1955, in comparison to a control population provided by the

Officers of the Metropolitan Police (177). An epidemiological survey monograph by Dr. Roberts was separately published with the report of the Committee on Boxing (40). Some of the affirmations and conclusions made by the Committee on Boxing in their report on the medical aspects of boxing were the following (177):

1. The prevailing evidence supports that "There is a danger of chronic brain damage occurring in boxers as a result of their careers."

2. "Boxers, by the nature of their sport, are liable to injury. In rare accidents this may result in acute severe brain damage, hemorrhage and even death. It had not been suggested until recently that what seemed to be a comparatively mild injury to the head, causing only a short lived disturbance of function, might lead to cumulative and permanent damage to the delicate tissues of the nervous system if often repeated."

3. The prevalence of the clinical signs and evidence of brain damage in retired boxers increases with increasing exposure to boxing.

4. "The hazards inherent in the sport will, however, remain and it is probable that prolonged exposure to them will continue to carry with it the likelihood of some degree of permanent injury to the brain."

5. "Many professional boxers know of colleagues who, as a result of their careers, have developed a chronic disabling condition, which they call 'punch drunk'....In a number of these well documented cases the condition appeared to have progressed despite the retirement of the boxer from the ring."

6. Most of the sufferers of the punch drunk state dated the onset of their symptoms to the end of their boxing careers, when they were relatively young, and thought that their disabilities had gradually progressed. Slurred speech, slowness and clumsiness of movement, unsteadiness of gait and tremors were the commonest features, while dementia occurred in about 20% of sufferers.

7. "Most of those affected had developed their disabilities towards the end of their boxing career. In a few cases the condition appeared to have become more obvious, especially to the wives, as the boxers had grown older," and appeared to have advanced more rapidly and earlier than could have been accounted for by normal aging alone. There was no evidence that boxing may have contributed or aggravated any other systemic disease found in boxers. Boxers "who were found to be severely affected suffered from slurring of speech to the point of being almost unintelligible, defective memory and slow thought. In some the limbs were stiff, the face expressionless, their walk a slow shuffle and their body and hands affected by a tremor at rest."

8. The presence of defects in the septum pellucidum on air-encephalography of boxers was not considered in itself to be responsible for the clinical picture of chronic brain damage, but confirmed the presence of structural brain damage, almost certainly due to boxing (178-180). The examined brains of boxers showed evidence of cerebral atrophy, ragged holes in the septum pellucidum, extensive loss of neurons in the cerebral cortex and brainstem nuclei responsible for control of voluntary movement and neurofibrillary degeneration of cells as seen in brains of old people or sufferers of progressive dementia in middle life. The frequency of epilepsy in boxers when compared to the general population was not increased. And the diagnosis of traumatic encephalopathy in boxers should not rely exclusively on a single medical or radiologic finding.

9. 17% [one in six] of examined boxers showed evidence of damage to the nervous system attributable to boxing, and probably only one-third of these were so affected severely enough to be recognized as punch-drunk by a lay person. Two-thirds showed evidence of similar brain damage and manifested mild symptoms, which constituted an inconvenience to the sufferer, and seemed ap-

parent to a neurologist and possibly not apparent to a lay person.

10. The prevalence of brain damage increased with increasing occupational exposure to boxing measured by the length of professional career, number of professional fights and/or age at retirement. Among retired professional boxers aged 50 years and above, 47% of those who boxed for more than 10 years, 17% of those who boxed for six to nine years, and 13% of those who boxed for five years or less, showed evidence of brain damage. For younger professional boxers, the rates were 25%, 14% and 1% respectively. Sparing boxing partners who were engaged in boxing over long periods were more likely to have evidence of brain damage. Boxers in heavier [welterweight and above] than lighter classes [lightweight and below] were more likely to have evidence of brain damage. However, in every class of boxing, the longer the exposure to boxing, the higher the frequency of brain damage.

11. Severe acute brain injury, which may result in death is rare in both professional and amateur boxing (181); however a high mortality is associated with intracranial hemorrhages, which may occur rarely.

12. The committee recommended that all forms of competitive boxing should be supervised by organizations that were able to undertake responsibility for the medical welfare of boxers, and continuing personal records of all boxers engaged in competitive boxing should be maintained and possibly studied by the Royal College of Physicians.

In his 1969 book "Brain Damage in Boxers"(40), Roberts had asserted that Martland's 1928 paper (2) was the first report in the medical literature identifying boxing as a cause of chronic neurological disease. Martland had suggested that boxing as a definitive cause of punch drunk can be validated only by collection and analysis of statistical and neuropathological data, which Roberts and the Royal College of Physicians of London performed and reported by 1969. As part of his epidemiological study of boxers, Roberts performed a review of previously published reports on traumatic encephalopathy and was able to identify twenty-six case reports of traumatic encephalopathy in boxers published between 1928 and 1967 (2, 132, 133, 145, 179, 180, 182-201). These reports described fifty-three cases of boxers with a neurological syndrome which was considered to be caused by their boxing careers. The ages of these boxers ranged from 16 to 63 years old, and only 10 [19%] of these boxers were above the age of 50 years old. In addition to these case reports, Roberts reported three additional studies of boxers in Italy (202, 203), Germany (204) and Czechoslovakia (205, 206), which had supported the concept that a proportion of amateur and professional boxers developed severe neurological syndromes caused by boxing. Roberts also identified thirteen other published reports on traumatic encephalopathy in boxers (3, 146, 207-217), which he thought did not provide additional or adequately substantiated recorded data that would be used to support or refute the concept of CTE attributable to boxing. However, Roberts actually identified a paper by Kaplan and Browder (141) and the New York State Boxing Commission, published in the United States in 1954, which has been described above, asserting that there was no evidence that CTE was caused by boxing.

In his conclusions, Roberts stated that his study of professional boxers supported the implications of the data derived from other forms of head injury that comparatively minor head injury in man may produce permanent damage to cerebral tissue. Such damage can occur even without prolonged unconsciousness. In reference to professional boxers, he stated that prolonged exposure to the occupational trauma of boxing is in most cases necessary before clinical symptoms of neurological damage and impairment will manifest. The eventual clinical syndrome that develops is a result of the cumulative sum total of repeated minor lesions in cerebral tissue, each of negligible importance in terms of permanent impairment of neurological function. This syndrome would resemble that caused by one episode of severe head trauma with diffuse axonal injury, and both syndromes are likely to possess the same neuropathology (40).

Following the conclusions and recommendations of the Committee on Boxing (177) of the Royal College of Physicians of London in 1969 there followed an increasing consensus that repetitive traumatic brain injury in boxers can cause permanent brain damage and result in DP (218). It also became increasingly recognized that similar repetitive traumatic brain injury or concussions can also cause permanent brain damage and result in chronic brain injury or CTE in other types of contact sports (59, 218-222) including soccer (223-234), American football (44, 45, 235-238), ice hockey (239), wrestling and martial arts (7). Such permanent brain damage will result in a constellation of progressive neurological and neuropsychiatric symptomatology (218, 240). Dr. Barry Jordan of the brain injury program of the Burke Rehabilitation Hospital, White Plains, New York is one of the individuals who have done the most extensive work on DP (240). In a review paper he published in 2001 with Ribadi, Jordan (218) concluded that "Chronic traumatic brain injury has been well described in boxing. However, chronic traumatic brain injury can be anticipated in any contact sport [e.g., soccer, football, ice hockey, and the martial arts) where there is a risk of multiple subconcussive and concussive blows to the head". He further opined that the symptoms of chronic traumatic brain injury, including motor, cognitive, and behavioral impairments are delayed and often occur long after the cessation of a career and "the early diagnosis and documentation of neurologic dysfunction among active athletes can provide the necessary information that will enable medical supervisors to limit an athlete's exposure to further brain injury" (218).

HISTORICAL REPORTS ON THE NEUROPATHOLOGY OF CTE

Many published reports on the neuropathology of CTE in boxers prior to 1969 concerned brain lesions that were immediately relevant to the cause of death, most prevalently acute subdural hemorrhage (40). In his 1968 paper, Oppenheimer (138) demonstrated four diffuse microscopic neuropathologic changes following survival for more than twelve hours in brains of 59 deceased individuals who suffered all types of brain trauma from mild concussion to virtual decerebration. These diffuse changes comprised [1] anoxic cell injury; [2] multiple capillary hemorrhages, which were indistinguishable from gross vascular markings of cerebral parenchymal congestion; [3] microscopic disruption of nervous tissue and white matter tract degeneration by silver impregnation, which was not identified grossly; and [4] microglial reaction. He attributed these diffuse changes to acceleration injuries of the brain and concluded that they were seen in both trivial concussions and severe brain trauma. He suggested that further detailed studies of the topographic distributions of these microscopic changes will facilitate better understanding of acceleration injuries of the brain. Following brain trauma, Oppenheimer identified microglial activation beginning at about 15 hours post-trauma, becoming more pronounced at 24 to 48 hours post-trauma. He also identified axonal retraction balls accompanying clusters of activated microglia after about 48 hours post-trauma, as well as microscopic foci of pallor demonstrated by myelin stains. Activated microglia and histiocytes remained pronounced even at 2 weeks following trauma, and at about three weeks reactive astrocytes were seen. Pronounced microglial activation, histiocytes and activated astrocytes remained present even at 6 weeks following trauma. In patients who survived for months and years, microglial and astrocytic activation remained present constituting the major features of the trauma at this time. These changes were also noted in five cases of clinically trivial brain injuries involving concussions (138).

In 1956 and 1961, Strich (241, 242) reported brain degeneration and post-traumatic dementia following uncomplicated head injury in 20 patients who died from two days to 24 months after sustaining head injury. A majority of these patients had no fractures of the skull, no intracranial hemorrhages, and no large lacerations of the brain. Their brains showed diffuse white matter degeneration and demyelination admixed with axonal retraction bulbs, histiocytes and activated astrocytes. The cortex showed slight generalized neuronal loss accompanied by other gross findings of focal cortical contusions and scattered remote white matter micro-hemorrhages. Ventriculomegaly and/or necrotic foci were present in some cases. Strich's findings of white matter degeneration correlated with previously reported case reports of white matter degeneration following concussions in deceased brain trauma patients by Rosenblath [1899] and Meyer [1904]. Earlier, Russell [1932] and Greenfield [1938], had stressed the interruption of nerve function and nerve fibers by mechanical damage brought about by concussions; while Rand and Courville [1934] found retraction axonal bulbs in areas of the brain surrounding hemorrhages and contusions, as well as in areas remote from focal lesions, further generating tissue evidence linking concussions to white matter and nerve fiber damage. Strich (241, 242) in his conclusion stated that the shear stresses and strains of rotational acceleration of the head from blunt force trauma caused tearing or stretching of nerve fibers, which resulted in secondary diffuse white matter degeneration that followed concussions and uncomplicated head injury, which consequently may permanently incapacitate the patient and result in dementia. However Strich could not determine if and when this white matter degeneration would become irreversible following trauma, and what role it played in the generation of signs and symptoms of dementia and concussions. Using high-speed cinematography in monkeys subjected to blows to the head, Pudenz and Shelden (243), in 1946, generated evidence showing gliding and swirling movements of the brain, even after minor subconcussive blows, causing angular acceleration of the brain. If the head was free to move, these movements of the brain were greater than if the head was fixed.

Brandenburg and Hallervorden [1954] (194) were the first to report frequent "senile" plaques in the atrophic cortex of a 51 year old deceased punch-drunk boxer who had boxed as an amateur for eleven years and became a German middle-weight champion. Ten years after his retirement, when he was 38 years old, he became forgetful and excitable with a vague speech. In the year before his death he developed obvious signs of a parkinsonian syndrome with dementia. He eventually died from intracerebral hemorrhage at the age of 51 years old without arteriosclerosis or hypertension. The brain showed cortical atrophy with many neurofibrillary tangles [fibrillary degeneration of nerve cells] and senile plaques, accentuated in the frontal cortex, resembling the plaques seen in "senile dementia", "Alzheimer's Psychosis" or AD (38, 133), accompanied by amyloid vascular degeneration [vasculopathy]. The brain also showed scattered loss of Purkinje neurons, mild loss of nigral neurons with many of the residual nigral neurons showing Alzheimer's type neurofibrillary tangles. Based on their case report, Brandenburg and Hallervorden (194) reaffirmed that repetitive trauma to the head as seen in boxing does have the same effect as a single episode of head injury, which occasionally precipitates the onset of AD. They opined that their case was that of a special form of post-traumatic dementia with parkinsonism and delayed traumatic apoplexy (38).

Between Cassaca [1924] (176), Osnato and Giliberti [1927] (14), Martland and Beling [1927] (244), there were a total of 414 autopsied brains in individuals who died after sustaining concussions. Martland and Beling described "multiple miliary hemorrhages" or "multiple concussion hemorrhages", which were not immediately related to the traumatic focus. They had expounded the work of Bauchet [1860], Gowers [1888], Walz [1896] and Bailey [1909] who had earlier propounded the underlying mechanisms of concussions in relation to permanent brain damage (244). Bauchet proposed oscillatory movements of the head as a mechanism of concussions, when the oscillations were transferred to the brain causing an insult to brain tissue that produced considerable derangement of the molecules of the brain. Intuitively, Bauchet had recognized that the brain can resist external violence under certain conditions and will not develop any visible or appreciable alteration. Also Morgagni (244) had intuited as a mechanism of concussions that during head trauma, the brain is driven against the skull and at the same time repelled by the skull, subjecting the brain to two motions in opposite directions, and if the skull is not fractured, the entire forces of percussion are directed against the brain itself. Bauchet went further to delineate brain concussion [commotion] from brain contusion indicating that concussions were more diffuse and comprised vascular congestion with or without small miliary extravasations without physical disruption of the brain substance. In contusions, the brain substance was physically altered and the damage was more limited and more profound and involved an admixture of hemorrhages and brain substance (244). Gowers, in addition, opined that the hemorrhages seen in the brain following concussions were due to the slight support given by cerebral tissues to the cerebral blood vessels, and the traumatic consequences of concussions could produce delayed paralysis agitans by the concussion of nerve centers in the brain. Bailey later reaffirmed Gowers' proposition that there was a causal relationship between the injury of concussions and brain trauma, and traumatic paralysis agitans as a disease. Intuitively though, Walz had suspected that this disease appeared only in people with previous deterioration of the nervous system, a deterioration that may as well have been caused by prior concussions or brain injuries (244).

In 1929 Martland (244) reported their findings in 309 autopsies he performed over a two year period as chief medical examiner of Essex County, New Jersey, on persons dying of cerebral injuries exclusive of gunshot and penetrating force wounds of the head. Out of this cohort, Martland (244) reported only nine cases [2.9%] of multiple, small, discrete, punctate and sometimes confluent parenchymal hemorrhages of the cerebral white matter and gray matter of the basal nuclei. These hemorrhages were the only gross evidence of brain injury. There was no cortical cerebral contusion or laceration, and no fracture of the skull [except in one case, which showed negligible fracture of the supra-orbital plate of the frontal bone]. There were no hemorrhages in the cerebellum or brainstem, except in one case, which showed small hemorrhages in the rostral cervical spinal medulla (244). Microscopically, these lesions comprised marked vascular congestion of the penetrating parenchymal blood vessels with perivascular microextravasates.

Martland termed these hemorrhages "concussion hemorrhages" and opined that they were similar to the hemorrhages reported by Cassasa (176) in his five cases, and that these hemorrhages practically never occured when the calvarium of the skull was fractured. Martland also identified traumatic fat embolism as a possible differential diagnosis for concussion hemorrhages. However, they concluded that concussion hemorrhages may occur in mild concussions of the brain and may persist in less vital regions of the brain without causing symptoms. In more severe concussions, these hemorrhages initiated inflammatory tissue responses in the brain, which would form the basis of the symptomatology of postconcussion neuroses or psychoses (244). They further concluded that injuries of the brain may occur with slight or no external evidence of injuries, comprising only concussion hemorrhages, which may result in death in a certain percentage of cases or in persistent clinical symptoms indicating structural damage to the brain. Their final conclusion was: "Every case of injury to the head should be considered serious, and the patient should receive careful neurologic examination and observation, as an apparently trivial head injury may be followed by grave results and may be of great importance to civil and workmen's compensation courts in the estimation of disabilities and the assessment of damages" (244).

Cassasa (176) in 1924 reported multiple and punctate cerebral parenchymal hemorrhages in five autopsied decedents from the New York Medical Examiner's office who died following head trauma without any lacerations of the scalp, fractures of the skull, cortical lacerations or contusions, except occasional pial hemorrhages. He found only five of these cases over a ten year period of work with the chief medical examiner of New York County and thought it to be relatively rare. He had opined that these peculiar types of multiple traumatic cerebral hemorrhages were rare and possibly explained the pathology and injury mechanism of concussions of the brain. The hemorrhages were perivascular and either limited to the Virchow Robin spaces or to the brain matter immediately adjoining the blood vessels. Cassasa propounded that the occurrence of these hemorrhages showed that concussion of the brain was a more permanent injury condition, which depended upon the number and extent of these hemorrhages, and may form the basis of the prolonged sequelae of concussions.

In their quest to identify a structural basis for post-traumatic psychoneurosis and link it to concussion, Osnato and Giliberti (14) examined 100 cases of concussion of the brain with or without fracture of the skull. Their patients had sustained blunt force traumas of the head and were claimants for damages for their injuries under compensation and liability laws. Thirty-two of the 100 patients did not show any wound to the scalp, or any fracture of the skull. Osnato and Giliberti (14) concluded by refuting Trotter's definition of concussion as a transient state, which did not comprise any structural damage to the brain. They affirmed that concussions comprise actual injuries to the brain and in a proportion of cases, complete resolution does not occur resulting in secondary degenerative changes or post-concussion neurosis.

Payne's (245) 1968 paper titled "Brains of boxers" enumerated the neuropathological findings in six deceased retired professional boxers. The symptomatology common to all cases included, but were not limited to chronic alcoholism, manic depressive psychosis, depression, compulsive gambling, violent behavior, emotional lability, paranoia, insomnia, marital disharmony, inability to remain employed for long durations, headaches, memory impairment, impaired concentration, confusion, intellectual deterioration, confusion, dysarthria and ataxia. The prevalent neuropathological findings in all cases included but were not limited to leptomeningeal thickening, slight to moderate cerebral atrophy, some enlargement of the ventricular system, fenestrations of the septum pellucidum and presence of cavum septi pellucidi, multifocal cortical scarring and gliosis with minimal to mild cortical neuronal dropout, multifocal cortical white matter and myelin degeneration, chronic inflammation with perivascular lymphocytes and pigment-laden and foamy histiocytes, neuropil histiocytes, as well as a small number of cortical and hippocampal senile amyloid plaques in only one case, and early neurofibrillary changes in only two cases. Payne concluded that there was little doubt that the brain disturbances, which sometimes occurred in ex-boxers were in part, at least, due to the lesions he observed in his cohort of six deceased retired boxers (245).

Earlier in 1957, Graham and Ule (134) had reported cortical cerebral atrophy with ventriculomegaly in the brain of a deceased 48 year old retired boxer who had developed progressive parkinsonian symptoms and dementia approximately ten years after his retirement at the age of 25 years old, after a ten year career. He was noted to have developed by the age of 46 years old, what was described as dull-euphoric dementia, with poorly defined focal symptoms, extrapyramidal disturbances, and progressive external and internal hydrocephalus. He died as a result of hemorrhagic infarction of the right frontal and parietal lobes due to thrombosis of the dural sinuses and meningeal veins. Brain histology confirmed neuronal loss with neurofibrillary tangles in the neocortex, subcortical ganglia and brainstem nuclei. There were no amyloid senile plaques in any region of the brain. Old contusions were absent (134). Graham and Ule recommended that cases like their case manifesting chronic progressive neurologic disorders after a symptom-free interval be termed DP, while cases manifesting neurologic disturbances in immediate connection with head injuries be termed traumatic encephalopathy of boxers (197).

Neubuerger (197) reported two additional cases of DP in 1959 when he described the neuropathological findings in a cortical brain biopsy and in an autopsied whole brain in two retired middle aged boxers who suffered from DP. The whole brain showed cortical brain atrophy, ventriculomegaly, mild to moderate cortical neuronal loss with astrogliosis, cortical white matter astrogliosis accentuated around the blood vessels, cortical white matter fiber loss and demyelination, neuronal loss in the presubiculum of the hippocampus and mild loss of the cerebellar internal granule neurons. The brain biopsy showed mild cortical neuronal loss, fibrillary astrogliosis, neurofibrillary tangles and senile plaques. No tangles or plaques were noted in the whole brain. Based on these two cases, Neubuerger inferred that "It is conceivable that multiple, partly subliminal concussions, repeated over a period of years, produce an altered state of the cerebral colloids, with inability to revert to the normal equilibrium. This process leads to precocious aging of the colloids" (197).

Corsellis (38) in 1973 published characteristic patterns of brain changes observed over a period of sixteen years in the brains of 15 retired boxers who suffered from symptoms of DP or punch drunk syndrome. Their ages at death ranged from 57 to 91 years old with a mean of 69 years old. Based on their review and findings in the individual cases, Corsellis (38) surmised that the following changes may be characteristic findings in brains of DP sufferers outside telltale signs of post-traumatic encephalopathy, focal and lobar cerebral contusions, lacerations and necrosis: fenestrations of the septum pellucidum, prominent or enlarged cavum septi pellucidi and cavum vergae; inferior cerebellar cortical astrogliosis and atrophy, neuronal loss and demyelination of the subcortical folial white matter, accentuated in the tonsillar regions; hypopigmentation of the substantia nigra and locus ceruleus with neuronal loss and neurofibrillary tangles in many residual neurons without Lewy bodies; non-AD topographic pattern of neurofibrillary tangles, diffusely spread in the neocortex and brainstem, accentuated in the mesial temporal lobe and amygdala, temporal, frontal and insular cortex, relatively sparing the parietal and occipital lobes, and accompanied by none to sparse senile amyloid plaques. Other frequent findings were brain atrophy and loss of volume of cerebral hemispheres, atrophy of the corpus callosum, ventriculomegaly of the lateral and third ventricles, varying degrees of mild to severe topographic neuronal loss and varying degrees of cerebral white matter pallor, demyelination and astrogliosis. In addition to these prevailing neuropathologic changes, Corsellis (38) noted the following symptoms that were common to their cohort: alcohol abuse, rage reactions, memory impairment, memory loss, and dementia. Although they did not denote their findings with any specific name or disease entity, Corsellis (38) concluded that the paramount reason for the insidious neurological and psychological deterioration in their cohort of boxers was brain damage incurred from boxing, for destroyed cerebral tissue could never be replaced and the process of degeneration could smolder on even after the boxer stopped boxing. In their paper, they also mentioned several researchers who had mentioned neuropathologic findings in sufferers of dementia following head injury (179, 246, 247), whose cases were included in their cohort of fifteen boxers except the case reported by Constantinides and Tissot (247) who had described similar findings in a 58 year old deceased retired boxer. After his retirement, he had developed mental deterioration, progressive intellectual and memory deterioration, behavioral impairment and parkinsonism with occasional epileptic attacks. His brain was moderately atrophied, a cavum septi pellucidi with fenestrations was present, the substantia nigra was hypopigmented, and a cortical micro-scar was noted in the left superior frontal sulcus. Abundant neurofibrillary tangles were noted in the mesial temporal lobe, substantia nigra, locus ceruleus and periventricular nuclei (38, 247).

With advent and evolution of immunohistochemical tissue technology in the 1980's and 1990's, there were many case reports, case series, and animal studies reporting the neuropathology of DP with the immunohistochemical identification and confirmation of abnormal protein accumulations. In 1996, Geddes et al (16) reported a unique immunophenotype of isolated taupathy in a 23 year old professional boxer who began boxing at the age of eleven years. Computerized tomography scans of his brain had been normal; however, he was described to be somewhat forgetful. He had died days after sustaining a subdural hemorrhage from a fight. At autopsy, his brain appeared grossly within normal limits except for congestive brain swelling and cerebral edema with mass effect, transtentorial and transforaminal cerebral herniation accompanied by brainstem herniation [Duret] hemorrhages. His brain did not show brain atrophy or any other gross evidence of brain damage (16). Histologically, there was evidence of his terminal acute brain trauma with excitotoxic neuronal injury and focal axonal injury in the splenium of the corpus callosum. No neocortical neuronal loss was detected, and no obvious cell loss of the cerebellar cortex, locus ceruleus, and substantia nigra was present. No cerebral or cerebellar cortical scarring was seen. The principal histomorphologic and immunophenotypic findings were tau-immunopositive neocortical neurofibrillary tangles and neuritic threads, which were accentuated in the inferolateral surfaces of the brain, fusiform gyrus, inferior temporal, middle frontal and orbital gyri, with focal collections in the supramarginal gyrus of the parietal cortex and the frontal cortex. Very rare tangles were found in the occipital cortex and cingulum. The tangles were distributed in all layers of the neocortex in a patchy fashion and appeared to be closely associated and grouped around penetrating parenchymal blood vessels. Uniquely, there were no tangles or neuritic threads in the mesial temporal cortex, including the amygdala and hippocampal complex [dentate fascia, cornu ammonis, subiculum, transentorhinal and entorhinal cortex], other subcortical nuclei and brainstem nuclei. Just one tangle was found in the nucleus basalis of Meynert. There was no astrogliosis associated with the tangles. Geddes et al (16) revolutionized CTE with this case report, near-completely changing the way this disease had been envisioned and characterized. They concluded that "In the absence of other disease, it appears that in this young boxer neurofibrillary tangles were the result of repeated head injury, and the earliest signs of chronic traumatic brain damage. Their preponderance at the anatomical sites at which contusions are characteristically found suggests that their formation may have been related to impact and resultant tissue damage" (16).

In 1999, Geddes et al (51) published yet another epoch-making paper describing the immunophenotypic changes in the brain following mild head injury in five young men between the ages of 23 and 28 years old comprising two boxers, one soccer player, one mentally subnormal man with a history of head banging and an epileptic who repeatedly hit his head during seizures. Again, their brains did not show the expected evidence of physical brain damage caused by repetitive chronic brain trauma. Rather, there were only histological changes comprised of tau-immunopositive neocortical neurofibrillary tangles which were occasionally solitary in some areas and numerous in some areas, strikingly arranged in groups, sited predominantly around small intracortical blood vessels (51). Neuropil neuritic threads were also present. The basal surfaces of the brain were most affected, often in the depths of the sulci, around blood vessels, involving all layers of the neocortex. There was no perivascular astrocytosis or microglial proliferation. The hippocampus was not involved and appeared normal except in a single case which showed a focus of neurofibrillary tangles around a blood vessel in the transentorhinal cortex. No amyloid plaques were found in any of the five cases. Interestingly, Geddes et al (51) were able to determine the apolipoprotein E [ApoE] genotype of two of their cases, and both cases turned out to be have the E3/E3 ApoE genotype (51). Geddes et al finally concluded that "What is clear from our study of these five cases is that chronic mild repetitive head injury, such as that sustained by boxers, leads at any early age to subclinical but definable pathological changes, observable as neurofibrillary tangles in the absence of beta-amyloid peptide and with a strong suggestion of a causal association with vessels" (51).

Earlier in 1988, Roberts (248) re-examined eight brains from the cohort of retired professional boxers reported by Corsellis (38), using immunohistochemistry. Roberts identified the presence of predominantly tau-immunopositive neurofibrillary tangles with or without amyloid plaques. Amyloid plaques were rarely present, and, when present, were much smaller in number, less obvious, and comprised the primitive types of plaques with no plaque cores. Neurofibrillary tangles were present in the hippocampus, subiculum and temporal cortex. They were found predominantly in pyramidal neurons as well as in smaller neurons and in all layers of the lateral temporal cortex, though limited to the outer layers in the medial temporal cortex [parahippocampal gyrus and uncus]. Roberts (248) concluded that the prevailing evidence "...strongly supported the idea that head injury and its associated brain trauma may be one of the several predisposing factors in the process of tangle formation".

However, in a later paper in 1990, using newly developed

immunohistochemical methods for amyloid-beta protein, Roberts (249) identified the presence of diffuse amyloid plaques in the temporal cortex of fourteen of the fifteen cases reported by Corsellis (38). Roberts noted that the tangles and plaques seen in cases of DP resemble those seen in AD, and concluded that head injury causing neuronal shearing and/or damage to the vascular system may precipitate the pathological processes, which give rise to AD (249). As part of the foundational evidence for his conclusion, Roberts referenced a case report by Rudelli (250) which had described progressive dementia in a 38 year old man who had suffered a single episode of severe traumatic brain injury 16 years earlier, sustained from an automobile crash when he was only 22 years old, and recovered substantially following surgical interventions. Several years after his injury, he began to exhibit personality changes with greater docility, behavioral changes with impulsive outbursts, and absenteeism from work. He exhibited regression in intellectual functioning, got separated from his family, and lost his job. His speech became reduced to single words and phrases, but he followed simple directions. He eventually experienced urinary incontinence and myoclonic jerking of his trunk and extremities aggravated by intentional movement, and only walked with the assistance of two people. Computerized tomography scans of the head revealed cortical atrophy with ventriculomegaly. With his continued decline he was hospitalized, became bedridden and mute, with flexion contractures requiring feeding gastrostomy. He eventually died from septicemia with bronchopneumonia and urinary tract infection. His brain revealed diffuse cortical atrophy and weighed only 1050 grams. There were focal old contusions in the frontal and temporal lobes. The cerebellum and brainstem appeared normal except for focal lateral old contusions of the left cerebellar hemisphere. The corpus callosum was atrophic and the septum pellucidum showed no fenestrations. The third and lateral ventricles were dilated. The substantia nigra was not pale. The hippocampus was atrophic. Histology revealed abundant numbers of neurofibrillary tangles and neuritic amyloid plaques in the neocortex, subcortical ganglia and brainstem ganglia. Rudelli opined that the subject in his case report suffered from a post-traumatic dementia (250).

Using histochemical and immunohistochemical stains, in 1990, Allsop (251) examined the temporal lobes of six of the original fifteen cases reported by Corsellis (38) in addition to two cases of retired boxers aged 22 to 77 years old. They found diffuse amyloid plaques [7 of 8 cases] and sparse to frequent neurofibrillary tangles [6 of 8 cases]. No plaques or tangles were noted in the 22 year old ex-boxer. Neurofibrillary tangles were not seen in a 58 year old boxer, but moderate amyloid plaques were noted. In 1991, Tokuda (252) again examined the temporal lobes of seven of the original fifteen cases reported by Corsellis (38), and one additional case of a retired boxer, all aged 56 to 83 years old, using histochemical and immunohistochemical stains. They found frequent neurofibrillary tangles in the neocortex [8 of 8 cases] accompanied by neuritic neuropil threads [7 of 8 cases], senile amyloid plaques [8 of 8 cases] and amyloid deposits on the meningeal and penetrating parenchymal cerebral blood vessels [3 of 8 cases]. Tokuda (252) and Allsop (251) concluded that the pathological findings in DP resembled the findings in AD and that these diseases may share common etiological and pathogenic mechanisms especially in relation to trauma.

Parallel to the studies in human brains, there have also been empirical studies in animal models exploring the neuropathology of the sequelae of chronic and repetitive traumatic brain injuries (253-256). In testing whether brain trauma has prolonged effects and initiates insidiously progressive neurodegenerative processes, Smith (254) in 1999, used traumatic pig models to demonstrate post-traumatic axonal bulbs and swellings, as well as accumulation of beta amyloid protein and tau protein in the brains of pigs exposed to diffuse traumatic axonal injury, one to ten days post-trauma. Beta amyloid was only found in one-third of the pigs who had the highest total amount of axonal pathology (254). Earlier in 1997, Smith (257) had demonstrated progressive cortical and subcortical brain atrophy with ventriculomegaly, neuronal loss and astrogliosis in rats up to one year after fluid-percussion traumatic brain injury. Smith concluded that there was a link between brain trauma and the initiation of chronic progressive neurodegenerative processes, and pathologic cascades of neuro-degenerative diseases may follow diffuse brain injury.

In 2002, Uryu (255) tested whether single or repetitive mild traumatic brain injury resulted in AD-like changes in the brain using a mouse model of mild traumatic brain injury. They found that single and repetitive mild traumatic brain injury in mice resulted in astrogliosis in the cortex, hippocampus, subcortical white matter, and corpus callosum. Accumulation of beta amyloid protein was observed in the brains of their mice models following both single and repetitive mild traumatic brain injury. Also, their mice models showed earlier, higher and more persistent evidence of oxidative stress following repetitive mild traumatic brain injury than single mild traumatic brain injury using levels of isoprostanes in the brain and urine as a marker of lipid peroxidation. Uryu (255) concluded that there was a clear positive correlation between episodes of traumatic brain injury and accumulation of amyloid in the brain, as well as cognitive impairment and lipid peroxidation. Both single and repetitive mild traumatic brain injuries induced pathologic changes in the brain; however, single episodes of mild traumatic brain injury induced a milder pathology than repetitive mild traumatic brain injury. They further concluded that their findings were strongly supportive of traumatic brain injury being one of the most robust environmental risk factors for AD.

Still using mouse models, Yoshiyama (256) in 2005 further demonstrated that mild repetitive traumatic brain injury can result in accumulation of neurofibrillary tangle-like inclusions and pathological species of tau in the brain accompanied by neurobehavioral impairment. However, out of a cohort of eighteen transgenic mice exposed to controlled cortical impacts, only one mouse exhibited neurobehavioral impairment and increased tau pathology. In addition to tau pathology, this mouse exhibited cortical atrophy and ventriculomegaly. Astrogliosis was also present without beta amyloid protein deposits. Having observed this phenomenon in only one mouse, Yoshiyama (256) postulated that mild repetitive traumatic brain injury may not routinely lead to accelerated neurofibrillary tangle formation and that additional factors may be involved in the induction of neurofibrillary tangle formation following mild repetitive traumatic brain injury. Interestingly, Yoshiyama (256) and Uryu (255) reported the presence of meningeal and neuropil iron deposits following single and repetitive traumatic brain injury. Yoshiyama opined that the presence of iron may facilitate the accumulation of neurofibrillary tangles as a source of damaging reactive oxygen species via the Fenton reaction when iron [II] is oxidized by hydrogen peroxide to iron [III] producing hydroxyl radicals [OH] (256).

In addition to animal studies, Roberts (6, 48, 49) and Graham (47) also reported that brain trauma outside sports can result in accumulation of AD-like beta amyloid protein in the brains of individuals who have suffered single or repetitive brain injury. In 1991, Roberts (48) examined the brains of sixteen patients aged 10 to 63 years old who sustained severe head injury and survived for only six to eighteen days. Using immunostains for beta-amyloid protein, they found the presence of neocortical diffuse amyloid plaques in six of the sixteen [38%] patients. Roberts concluded that severe head injury can trigger deposition of amyloid protein in the brain within days of the injury, probably brought about by induction of the amyloid precursor protein mRNA in the brain as a normal response to neuronal stress, a protective induction that can become a disease process in susceptible individuals (48). They opined that their neuropathological findings support that head injury is the most consistently associated environmental factor implicated in 2 – 20% of AD cases (258, 259).

Roberts (49) later expanded their study in 1994 to examine 152 patients aged 8 weeks to 81 years old who had suffered severe brain injury and survived for four hours to 2.5 years. This cohort confirmed the original finding that beta-amyloid deposits are found in one or more cortical areas of approximately one-third of severe brain injury survivors. Increased neuronal beta-amyloid precursor protein [βAPP] immunopositivity was also found in close proximity to the extracellular beta-amyloid deposits. Roberts (49) proposed that increased βAPP, as part of an acute phase response to neuronal injury in the human brain can lead to deposition of beta-amyloid and initiation of an AD-type process within days, and head injury can be an important etiological factor in AD. In their cohort, interestingly, no beta-amyloid deposition was seen in the brain of any head injury patient under the age of 10 years old. The medial temporal cortex was the area that was most often affected (49).

Graham (47) went further in 1995 to study and map the distribution of beta-amyloid in fourteen individuals aged less than 65 years old, who died after suffering severe non-missile brain injury and survived for 3 hours to 4.5 weeks. They confirmed that beta-amyloid is widely deposited in the neocortex following brain injury in the form of diffuse plaques in all fourteen cases, without any correlation with cerebral contusions, intracranial hemorrhage, axonal injury, ischemic brain damage, brain swelling or raised intracranial hemorrhage. There was no asymmetry between cerebral hemispheres and the deposits were always bilateral. There were equal amounts of deposits in the frontal, temporal, parietal and occipital lobes, and plaques were found only in gray matter, much less commonly in subcortical gray matter, than neocortical gray matter. Plaques were deposited in a random fashion throughout the cortex without any accentuation or localization related to anatomical pathways, focal or diffuse pathologies of traumatic brain injury. Plaques were found in the cerebellar cortex in only two cases, and no plaques were found in the midbrain and pons in all cases. They opined, therefore, that beta-amyloid deposition following brain injury is a consequence of acute phase response of neurons to stress in susceptible individuals and serves as a useful model for studying the molecular basis of AD (47).

Dekosky et al. (50) in 2007 further confirmed the findings of Roberts (48, 49) and Graham (47) when they quantified brain tissue levels of beta-amyloid peptide and the precursor protein in the brains of nineteen patients who suffered severe closed head injury outside sports in relation to beta-amyloid plaque formation. They used temporal cortex tissue removed during decompressive craniectomy to relieve intractable brain swelling. Beta-amyloid plaques were found in six of the patients and the mean interval between injury and tissue extraction for this group was 11.9 hours. They observed a trend toward a correlation of higher soluble beta-amyloid levels with greater beta-amyloid plaque load in patients who showed beta-amyloid plaques. Soluble beta-amyloid was significantly higher in the plaque-positive patients than in the plaque-negative patients (50). Dekosky (50) concluded that high brain tissue levels of soluble beta-amyloid peptides and the development of cortical beta-amyloid plaques may predispose a subset of individuals with a brain injury to develop AD.

SUMMARY AND CONCLUSION

Published reports of the medical and scientific communities across the centuries confirm that concussions and subconcussions, as scientific concepts, are very well established concepts in medicine and fall within the generally accepted principles and common knowledge of medicine and science. The assertions of the chairman and leading members of the NFL committee on brain injury (1, 155, 161, 170, 171, 173, 175) are unsupported by prevailing published reports and papers in medicine and science. Published reports do not back up the assertion that it is typical for physicians-in-training to not receive any lecture or any training on concussions while in medical school, residency or fellowship training, and they do not support the assertion that physician knowledge regarding concussions and subconcussions is only anecdotal based only on word-of-mouth experiences informally passed from physicians to physicians and from non-physicians to physicians. The literature counters the claim that concussions and subconcussions are safe injuries that do not cause any permanent brain damage or brain neurodegeneration. CTE has been recognized and known by many names across the centuries [Table 4]. Published reports do not support the claims that there are very few experts on concussions; that there is very little scientific medical information on concussions.

In two letters to the editor, the chairman and members of the NFL brain injury committee asserted that repetitive head impacts in football cannot cause CTE in American football players and that there is no evidence that CTE occurs in football players (170, 171). In yet another published scientific paper, the chairman and members of the NFL brain injury committee claimed that it was safer to return a concussed football player to play in the same game in which he suffered a concussion, since players who return to play following a concussion have fewer initial signs and symptoms than those removed from play (161). Published scientific reports beginning as far back as the 17th century B.C., across many centuries, do not support these assertions, and do confirm that concussions and subconcussions are serious brain injuries, which should be taken seriously and possess the capacity to cause brain damage, progressive neurodegeneration (CTE), and death.

Given that concussions and subconcussions are serious brain injuries that cause brain damage, a value propositional debate is emerging on whether children should be intentionally exposed to potential repeated concussions and subconcussions in contact sports, risking damage to their young developing brains. Fortunately, the American Academy of Pediatrics [AAP] (74) has undertaken a leadership role in this debate when they issued a policy statement in 2011 on boxing participation by children and adolescents, reaffirming that: "Concussions are one of the most common injuries that occur with boxing. Because of the risk of head and facial injuries, the American Academy of Pediatrics and the Canadian Paediatric Society oppose boxing as a sport for children and adolescents. These organizations recommend that physicians vigorously oppose boxing in youth and encourage patients to participate in alternative sports in which intentional head blows are not central to the sport." It is interesting to note that other medical organizations that have recommended the prohibition of boxing in children younger than 18 years old include the American Medical Association [2007], the Australian Medical Association [2007], the British Medical Association [2007] and the World Medical Association [2005] (74). The continuing question that arises in this debate based upon the recommendations of physicians across the world is: "What about other contact sports, outside boxing, in which intentional head blows are central to the sport?"

REFERENCES

1. Pellman EJ. Background on the National Football League's research on concussion in professional football. Neurosurgery 2003 Oct;53(4):797-8.

2. Martland HS. Punch Drunk. Journal of the American Medical Association 1928 October 13, 1928;91(15):1103-7.

3. Millspaugh JA. Dementia pugilistica. US Naval Medicine Bulletin 1937;35:297-303.

4. Omalu B. Play hard, die young : football depression, dementia, and death. 1st ed. Lodi, CA: Neo-Forenxis Books; 2008.

5. Omalu BI, DeKosky ST, Minster RL, Kamboh MI, Hamilton RL, Wecht CH. Chronic traumatic encephalopathy in a National Football League player. Neurosurgery 2005 Jul;57(1):128-34; discussion -34.

6. Roberts GW, Whitwell HL, Acland PR, Bruton CJ. Dementia in a punch-drunk wife. Lancet 1990 Apr 14;335(8694):918-9.

7. Aotsuka A, Kojima S, Furumoto H, Hattori T, Hirayama K. [Punch drunk syndrome due to repeated karate kicks and punches]. Rinsho Shinkeigaku 1990 Nov;30(11):1243-6.

8. Omalu BI, DeKosky ST, Hamilton RL, Minster RL, Kamboh MI, Shakir AM, et al. Chronic traumatic encephalopathy in a national football league player: part II. Neurosurgery 2006 Nov;59(5):1086-92; discussion 92-3.

9. Omalu BI, Hamilton RL, Kamboh MI, DeKosky ST, Bailes J. Chronic traumatic encephalopathy in a national football league player: case report and emerging medico-legal practice questions. . J Forensic Nurs 2010 Spring;6(1):40-6.

10. Omalu B, Bailes J, Hamilton RL, Kamboh MI, Hammers J, Case M, et al. Emerging histomorphologic phenotypes of chronic traumatic encephalopathy in American athletes. Neurosurgery Jul;69(1):173-83; discussion 83.

11. Omalu BI, Bailes J, Hammers JL, Fitzsimmons RP. Chronic Traumatic Encephalopathy, Suicides and Parasuicides in Professional American Athletes: The Role of the Forensic Pathologist. Am J Forensic Med Pathol 2009 June;31(2):130-2.

12. Omalu BI, Fitzsimmons RP, Hammers J, Bailes J. Chronic traumatic encephalopathy in a professional American wrestler. Journal of Forensic Nursing 2010;6(3):130-6.

13. Omalu B, Hammers JL, Bailes J, Hamilton RL, Kamboh MI, Webster G, et al. Chronic traumatic encephalopathy in an Iraqi war veteran with posttraumatic stress disorder who committed suicide. Neurosurg Focus Nov;31(5):E3.

14. Osnato M, Giliberti V. Postconcussion Neurosis-Traumatic Encephalitis. Arch Neurol and Psychiat 1927 August 1927;18:181-211.

15. Proceedings of the Congress of Neurological Surgeons in 1964. Report of the Ad Hoc Committee to Study Head Injury Nomenclature. Clin Neurosurg 1966;12:386-94.

16. Geddes JF, Vowles GH, Robinson SF, Sutcliffe JC. Neurofibrillary tangles, but not Alzheimer-type pathology, in a young boxer. Neuropathol Appl Neurobiol 1996 Feb;22(1):12-6.

17. Cervos-Navarro J, Lafuente JV. Traumatic brain injuries: structural changes. J Neurol Sci 1991 Jul;103 Suppl:S3-14.

18. Bigler ED. Neuropathology of acquired cerebral trauma. J Learn Disabil 1987 Oct;20(8):458-73.

19. Valsamis MP. Pathology of trauma. Neurosurg Clin N Am 1994 Jan;5(1):175-83.

20. Patt S, Brodhun M. Neuropathological sequelae of traumatic injury in the brain. An overview. Exp Toxicol Pathol 1999 Feb;51(2):119-23.

21. Adams JH, Graham DI, Jennett B. The structural basis of moderate disability after traumatic brain damage. J Neurol Neurosurg Psychiatry 2001 Oct;71(4):521-4.

22. Prince DA, Parada I, Scalise K, Graber K, Jin X, Shen F. Epilepsy following cortical injury: cellular and molecular mech-

anisms as targets for potential prophylaxis. Epilepsia 2009 Feb;50 Suppl 2:30-40.

23. Diaz-Arrastia R, Agostini MA, Madden CJ, Van Ness PC. Posttraumatic epilepsy: the endophenotypes of a human model of epileptogenesis. Epilepsia 2009 Feb;50 Suppl 2:14-20.

24. Dichter MA. Posttraumatic epilepsy: the challenge of translating discoveries in the laboratory to pathways to a cure. Epilepsia 2009 Feb;50 Suppl 2:41-5.

25. Pitkanen A, Immonen RJ, Grohn OH, Kharatishvili I. From traumatic brain injury to posttraumatic epilepsy: what animal models tell us about the process and treatment options. Epilepsia 2009 Feb;50 Suppl 2:21-9.

26. Hunt RF, Scheff SW, Smith BN. Posttraumatic epilepsy after controlled cortical impact injury in mice. Exp Neurol 2009 Feb;215(2):243-52.

27. Swartz BE, Houser CR, Tomiyasu U, Walsh GO, DeSalles A, Rich JR, et al. Hippocampal cell loss in posttraumatic human epilepsy. Epilepsia 2006 Aug;47(8):1373-82.

28. Statler KD. Pediatric posttraumatic seizures: epidemiology, putative mechanisms of epileptogenesis and promising investigational progress. Dev Neurosci 2006;28(4-5):354-63.

29. Povlishock JT, Katz DI. Update of neuropathology and neurological recovery after traumatic brain injury. J Head Trauma Rehabil 2005 Jan-Feb;20(1):76-94.

30. Graham DI, Adams JH, Nicoll JA, Maxwell WL, Gennarelli TA. The nature, distribution and causes of traumatic brain injury. Brain Pathol 1995 Oct;5(4):397-406.

31. Thom M, Liu JY, Thompson P, Phadke R, Narkiewicz M, Martinian L, et al. Neurofibrillary tangle pathology and Braak staging in chronic epilepsy in relation to traumatic brain injury and hippocampal sclerosis: a post-mortem study. Brain Oct;134(Pt 10):2969-81.

32. Khachaturian ZS. Diagnosis of Alzheimer's disease. Arch Neurol 1985 Nov;42(11):1097-105.

33. Khachaturian ZS. Diagnosis of Alzheimer's disease: two decades of progress. Alzheimers Dement 2005 Oct;1(2):93-8.

34. Khachaturian ZS. Diagnosis of Alzheimer's disease: two-decades of progress. J Alzheimers Dis 2006;9(3 Suppl):409-15.

35. Mirra SS, Hart MN, Terry RD. Making the diagnosis of Alzheimer's disease. A primer for practicing pathologists. Arch Pathol Lab Med 1993 Feb;117(2):132-44.

36. Hyman BT, Phelps CH, Beach TG, Bigio EH, Cairns NJ, Carrillo MC, et al. National Institute on Aging-Alzheimer's Association guidelines for the neuropathologic assessment of Alzheimer's disease. Alzheimers Dement Jan;8(1):1-13.

37. Mirra SS, Heyman A, McKeel D, Sumi SM, Crain BJ, Brownlee LM, et al. The Consortium to Establish a Registry for Alzheimer's Disease (CERAD). Part II. Standardization of the neuropathologic assessment of Alzheimer's disease. Neurology 1991 Apr;41(4):479-86.

38. Corsellis JA, Bruton CJ, Freeman-Browne D. The aftermath of boxing. Psychol Med 1973 Aug;3(3):270-303.

39. McKee AC, Cantu RC, Nowinski CJ, Hedley-Whyte ET, Gavett BE, Budson AE, et al. Chronic traumatic encephalopathy in athletes: progressive tauopathy after repetitive head injury. J Neuropathol Exp Neurol 2009 Jul;68(7):709-35.

40. Roberts AH. Brain damage in boxers. A study of the prevalence of traumatic encephalopathy among ex-professional boxers. London: Pitman Medical and Scientific Publishing Co.; 1969.

41. Amen DG, Newberg A, Thatcher R, Jin Y, Wu J, Keator D, et al. Impact of playing American professional football on long-term brain function. J Neuropsychiatry Clin Neurosci Fall;23(1):98-106.

42. Amen DG, Wu JC, Taylor D, Willeumier K. Reversing brain damage in former NFL players: implications for traumatic brain injury and substance abuse rehabilitation. J Psychoactive Drugs Jan-Mar;43(1):1-5.

43. Willeumier K, Taylor DV, Amen DG. Elevated body mass

in National Football League players linked to cognitive impairment and decreased prefrontal cortex and temporal pole activity. Transl Psychiatry;2:e68.

44. Guskiewicz KM, Marshall SW, Bailes J, McCrea M, Cantu RC, Randolph C, et al. Association between recurrent concussion and late-life cognitive impairment in retired professional football players. Neurosurgery 2005 Oct;57(4):719-26; discussion -26.

45. Guskiewicz KM, Marshall SW, Bailes J, McCrea M, Harding HP, Jr., Matthews A, et al. Recurrent concussion and risk of depression in retired professional football players. Med Sci Sports Exerc 2007 Jun;39(6):903-9.

46. McKee AC, Gavett BE, Stern RA, Nowinski CJ, Cantu RC, Kowall NW, et al. TDP-43 proteinopathy and motor neuron disease in chronic traumatic encephalopathy. J Neuropathol Exp Neurol Sep;69(9):918-29.

47. Graham DI, Gentleman SM, Lynch A, Roberts GW. Distribution of beta-amyloid protein in the brain following severe head injury. Neuropathol Appl Neurobiol 1995 Feb;21(1):27-34.

48. Roberts GW, Gentleman SM, Lynch A, Graham DI. beta A4 amyloid protein deposition in brain after head trauma. Lancet 1991 Dec 7;338(8780):1422-3.

49. Roberts GW, Gentleman SM, Lynch A, Murray L, Landon M, Graham DI. Beta amyloid protein deposition in the brain after severe head injury: implications for the pathogenesis of Alzheimer's disease. J Neurol Neurosurg Psychiatry 1994 Apr;57(4):419-25.

50. DeKosky ST, Abrahamson EE, Ciallella JR, Paljug WR, Wisniewski SR, Clark RS, et al. Association of increased cortical soluble abeta42 levels with diffuse plaques after severe brain injury in humans. Arch Neurol 2007 Apr;64(4):541-4.

51. Geddes JF, Vowles GH, Nicoll JA, Revesz T. Neuronal cytoskeletal changes are an early consequence of repetitive head injury. Acta Neuropathol 1999 Aug;98(2):171-8.

52. Armon C, Miller RG. Correspondence regarding: TDP-43 proteinopathy and motor neuron disease in chronic traumatic encephalopathy. J Neuropathol Exp Neurol 2010:69;918-29. J Neuropathol Exp Neurol Jan;70(1):97-8; author reply 8-100.

53. Bedlack RS, Genge A, Amato AA, Shaibani A, Jackson CE, Kissel JT, et al. Correspondence regarding: TDP-43 proteinopathy and motor neuron disease in chronic traumatic encephalopathy. J Neuropathol Exp Neurol 2010:69;918-29. J Neuropathol Exp Neurol Jan;70(1):96-7; author reply 8-100.

54. Chen-Plotkin AS, Lee VM, Trojanowski JQ. TAR DNA-binding protein 43 in neurodegenerative disease. Nat Rev Neurol Apr;6(4):211-20.

55. Armstrong RA, Ellis W, Hamilton RL, Mackenzie IR, Hedreen J, Gearing M, et al. Neuropathological heterogeneity in frontotemporal lobar degeneration with TDP-43 proteinopathy: a quantitative study of 94 cases using principal components analysis. J Neural Transm Feb;117(2):227-39.

56. Geser F, Lee VM, Trojanowski JQ. Amyotrophic lateral sclerosis and frontotemporal lobar degeneration: a spectrum of TDP-43 proteinopathies. Neuropathology Apr;30(2):103-12.

57. Uryu K, Nakashima-Yasuda H, Forman MS, Kwong LK, Clark CM, Grossman M, et al. Concomitant TAR-DNA-binding protein 43 pathology is present in Alzheimer disease and corticobasal degeneration but not in other tauopathies. J Neuropathol Exp Neurol 2008 Jun;67(6):555-64.

58. Neumann M, Sampathu DM, Kwong LK, Truax AC, Micsenyi MC, Chou TT, et al. Ubiquitinated TDP-43 in frontotemporal lobar degeneration and amyotrophic lateral sclerosis. Science 2006 Oct 6;314(5796):130-3.

59. Stern RA, Riley DO, Daneshvar DH, Nowinski CJ, Cantu RC, McKee AC. Long-term consequences of repetitive brain trauma: chronic traumatic encephalopathy. PM R Oct;3(10 Suppl 2):S460-7.

60. Robbins S. Doctors study link between combat and brain disease. Stars and Stripes. 2010 January 23, 2010.

61. Ropper A. Brain injuries from blasts. N Engl J Med 2011 Jun 2;364(22):2156-7.

62. Rosenfeld JV, Ford NL. Bomb blast, mild traumatic brain injury and psychiatric morbidity: a review. Injury 2010 May;41(5):437-43.

63. Goldstein LE, Fisher AM, Tagge CA, Zhang XL, Velisek L, Sullivan JA, et al. Chronic traumatic encephalopathy in blast-exposed military veterans and a blast neurotrauma mouse model. Sci Transl Med May 16;4(134):134ra60.

64. Ikonomovic MD, Uryu K, Abrahamson EE, Ciallella JR, Trojanowski JQ, Lee VM, et al. Alzheimer's pathology in human temporal cortex surgically excised after severe brain injury. Exp Neurol 2004 Nov;190(1):192-203.

65. Rovegno M, Soto PA, Saez JC, von Bernhardi R. [Biological mechanisms involved in the spread of traumatic brain damage]. Med Intensiva Jan-Feb;36(1):37-44.

66. Murayama S. [Seed, aggregation and propagation of abnormal proteins could explain neurodegeneration?]. Rinsho Shinkeigaku Nov;51(11):1097-9.

67. Polymenidou M, Cleveland DW. Prion-like spread of protein aggregates in neurodegeneration. J Exp Med May 7;209(5):889-93.

68. Nussbaum JM, Schilling S, Cynis H, Silva A, Swanson E, Wangsanut T, et al. Prion-like behaviour and tau-dependent cytotoxicity of pyroglutamylated amyloid-beta. Nature May 31;485(7400):651-5.

69. Guo JL, Lee VM. Seeding of normal Tau by pathological Tau conformers drives pathogenesis of Alzheimer-like tangles. J Biol Chem Apr 29;286(17):15317-31.

70. Baillargeon A, Lassonde M, Leclerc S, Ellemberg D. Neuropsychological and neurophysiological assessment of sport concussion in children, adolescents and adults. Brain Inj;26(3):211-20.

71. Franklin CC, Weiss JM. Stopping sports injuries in kids: an overview of the last year in publications. Curr Opin Pediatr Feb;24(1):64-7.

72. Field M, Collins MW, Lovell MR, Maroon J. Does age play a role in recovery from sports-related concussion? A comparison of high school and collegiate athletes. J Pediatr 2003 May;142(5):546-53.

73. Halstead ME, Walter KD. American Academy of Pediatrics. Clinical report--sport-related concussion in children and adolescents. Pediatrics Sep;126(3):597-615.

74. Purcell L, LeBlanc CM. Policy statement-Boxing participation by children and adolescents. Pediatrics Sep;128(3):617-23.

75. Karlin AM. Concussion in the pediatric and adolescent population: "different population, different concerns". PM R Oct;3(10 Suppl 2):S369-79.

76. Meehan WP, 3rd, Taylor AM, Proctor M. The pediatric athlete: younger athletes with sport-related concussion. Clin Sports Med Jan;30(1):133-44, x.

77. Bauer R, Fritz H. Pathophysiology of traumatic injury in the developing brain: an introduction and short update. Exp Toxicol Pathol 2004 Oct;56(1-2):65-73.

78. Anderson V, Moore C. Age at injury as a predictor of outcome following pediatric head injury: A longitudinal perspective. . Child Neuropsychology 1995;1(3):187-202.

79. Anderson V, Catroppa C, Morse S, Haritou F, Rosenfeld J. Functional plasticity or vulnerability after early brain injury? Pediatrics 2005 Dec;116(6):1374-82.

80. Li L, Liu J. The effect of pediatric traumatic brain injury on behavioral outcomes: a systematic review. Dev Med Child Neurol Sep 23.

81. Talavage TM, Nauman E, Breedlove EL, Yoruk U, Dye AE, Morigaki K, et al. Functionally-Detected Cognitive Impairment in High School Football Players Without Clinically-Diagnosed Concussion. J Neurotrauma Oct 1.

82. Herring SA, Cantu RC, Guskiewicz KM, Putukian M, Kibler WB, Bergfeld JA, et al. Concussion (mild traumatic brain injury) and the team physician: a consensus statement--2011 update. Med Sci Sports Exerc Dec;43(12):2412-22.

83. McCrory P, Meeuwisse W, Johnston K, Dvorak J, Aubry M, Molloy M, et al. Consensus statement on Concussion in Sport 3rd International Conference on Concussion in Sport held in Zurich, November 2008. Clin J Sport Med 2009 May;19(3):185-200.

84. Barkhoudarian G, Hovda DA, Giza CC. The molecular pathophysiology of concussive brain injury. Clin Sports Med Jan;30(1):33-48, vii-iii.

85. Aubry M, Cantu R, Dvorak J, Graf-Baumann T, Johnston KM, Kelly J, et al. Summary and agreement statement of the 1st International Symposium on Concussion in Sport, Vienna 2001. Clin J Sport Med 2002 Jan;12(1):6-11.

86. McCrory P, Johnston K, Meeuwisse W, Aubry M, Cantu R, Dvorak J, et al. Summary and agreement statement of the 2nd International Conference on Concussion in Sport, Prague 2004. Clin J Sport Med 2005 Mar;15(2):48-55.

87. Practice parameter: the management of concussion in sports (summary statement). Report of the Quality Standards Subcommittee. Neurology 1997 Mar;48(3):581-5.

88. Gronwall D, Wrightson P. Cumulative effect of concussion. Lancet 1975 Nov 22;2(7943):995-7.

89. Gronwall D, Wrightson P. Delayed recovery of intellectual function after minor head injury. Lancet 1974 Sep 14;2(7881):605-9.

90. Beiles D. In memoriam Prof. Dr. Milton Helpern. Z Rechtsmed 1977 Aug 26;80(2):170.

91. Sturner WQ. In memoriam: Milton Helpern, M.D. Am J Clin Pathol 1978 Jun;69(6):655.

92. Ward AA, Jr. The physiology of concussion. Clin Neurosurg 1964;12:95-111.

93. Littré A. Diverses observations anatomiques. Hist Acad Sci 1705:54-5.

94. Denny-Brown D. Brain trauma and concussion. Arch Neurol 1961 Jul;5:1-3.

95. Ommaya AK, Gennarelli TA. Cerebral concussion and traumatic unconsciousness. Correlation of experimental and clinical observations of blunt head injuries. Brain 1974 Dec;97(4):633-54.

96. Symonds C. Concussion and its sequelae. The Lancet 1962 January 6, 1962;1;7219(7219):1-5.

97. Brock S. Injuries of the skull, brain and spinal cord : neuro-psychiatric surgical and medico-legal aspects. Baillie\0300re Tindall and Cox: [s.n.]; 1940.

98. Miller GG. Cerebral Concussion. Archives of Surgery 1927 April 1927;14(4):891-916.

99. Trotter W. Certain Minor Injuries of the Brain. Lancet 1924 May 10, 1924;1:935.

100. Trotter W. ON CERTAIN MINOR INJURIES OF THE BRAIN: Being the Annual Oration, Medical Society of London. Br Med J 1924 May 10;1(3306):816-9.

101. Koch W, Filehne W. Beitrage zur experimentellen chirurgie: 3. ueber die commotio cerebri. . Arch f klin Chir 1874;17:190-231.

102. Schaller WF. After-effects of head injury: the post-traumatic concussion state (concussion, traumatic encephalopathy) and the post-traumatic psychoneurotic state (psychoneurosis, hysteria): a study in differential diagnosis. . The Journal of the American Medical Association 1939 November 11, 1939;113(20):1779-85.

103. Bell B. A System of Surgery. Edinburgh: C. Elliott; 1787.

104. Giza CC, Hovda DA. The Neurometabolic Cascade of Concussion. J Athl Train 2001 Sep;36(3):228-35.

105. Breasted JH. The Edwin Smith Surgical Papyrus. Chicago: University of Chicago Press; 1930.

106. Wilkins RH. Neurosurgical Classic. Xvii. J Neurosurg 1964 Mar;21:240-4.

107. Adams FS. The genuine works of Hippocrates. Translated ... with a preliminary discourse and annotations by F. Adams. London; 1849.

108. Strauss I, Savitsky N. Head injury, neurologic and psychiatric aspects. Archives of Neurology and Psychiatry 1934 May 1934;31(5):893-955.

109. Denny-Brown D, Russell WR. Experimental cerebral concussion. J Physiol 1940 Dec 20;99(1):153.

110. Denny-Brown D, Russell WR. Experimental Cerebral Concussion. Brain 1941 September, 1941;64:93-164.

111. Denny-Brown DE, Russell WR. Experimental Concussion: (Section of Neurology). Proc R Soc Med 1941 Sep;34(11):691-2.

112. Miles A. On the mechanism of brain injuries: preliminary considerations, various theories of concussion. Brain 1892;15(2):153-89.

113. Petit JL. Traité des maladies chirurgicales, et des opérations qui leur conviennent. Paris: Méquignon l'Aineé; 1790.

114. Cooper AP. Lectures on the principles and practice of surgery, with additional notes and cases by Frederick Tyrrel. Philadelphia: Haswell, Barrington & Haswell; 1839.

115. Boyer A. Traité des maladies chirurgicales, et des opérations qui leur conviennent. 3rd edition ed. Paris: Migneret; 1822.

116. Dupuytren G. Leçons orales de clinique chirurgicale faites â l'Hôtel-dieu de Paris. . 2nd edition ed. Paris: Germer-Baillière; 1839.

117. Erichsen JE. On concussion of the spine, nervous shock and other obscure injuries to the nervous system. New Edition ed. Baltimore: William Wood & Company; 1886.

118. Oppenheim H. Die traumatischen Neurosen nach den in der Nervenklinik der Charité in den 8 Jahren 1883-1891. 2nd Edition ed. Berlin: A. Hirschwald; 1892.

119. Horn P. Ueber Symptomatologie und Prognose der cerebralen Kommotionsneurosen unter vergleichender Berücksichtigung der Kopfkontusionen der Schädeldach-und Basisbrüche. Ztschr f d ges Neurol u Psychiat 1916;34:206.

120. Von Sarbó A. Granatenfernwirkungsfolgen und Kriegshysterie. Neurol Centralbl 1917;36:360.

121. Tromner E. Erinnerungen an die traumatische Hirnschwäche (Encephalopathia traumatica). Deutsche Ztschr f Nervenh 1921;68-69:491.

122. Russell WR. Cerebral involvement in head injury: a study based on the examination of 200 cases. Brain 1932;55(4):549-603.

123. Obersteiner H. Ueber Erschütterung des Rückenmarkes. Med Jahrb 1879:531.

124. Stevenson LD. Head injuries: effects and their appraisal: II. the role of the microglia. . Arch Neurol & Psychiat 1932;27(784).

125. Meyer A. The Anatomical Facts and Clinical Varieties of Traumatic Insanity. Am J Insan 1904 January 1904;6:374, 7, 82, 88.

126. Meyer A. The anatomical facts and clinical varieties of traumatic insanity, 1904. J Neuropsychiatry Clin Neurosci 2000 Summer;12(3):407-10.

127. Tanzi E, Lugaro E. Malattie Mentali. 2nd ed. Milan; 1914.

128. Peterson F, Haines WS, Webster RW. Legal Medicine and Toxicology. Saunders Company; 1923.

129. Oppenheim H. Die traumatischen neurosen. Berlin: Hirschwald; 1889.

130. Haase E. Bemerkenswerte pathologisch-anatomische befunde nach gehirnerschütterung. Zentralbl f d ges Neurol u Psychiat 1929-1930;54:637.

131. Bennet W. Some milder forms of concussion of the brain. In: Allbutt TC, Rolleston HD, editors. A system of medicine by many writers. London: The Macmillan Company; 1910. p. 231.

132. Critchley M. Punch drunk syndromes: the chronic traumatic encephalopathy of boxers. Hommage à Clovis Vincent. Paris: Maloine; 1949. p. 131.

133. Critchley M. Medical aspects of boxing, particularly from a neurological standpoint. Br Med J 1957 Feb 16;1(5015):357-62.

134. Graham H, Ule G. Beitrag zur kenntnis der chronischen cerebralen krankheitsbilder bei boxern. Psychiatria et Neurologiaii 1957;134:261-83.

135. Editorial: Brain damage in sport. Lancet 1976 Feb 21;1(7956):401-2.

136. Yarnell PR, Lynch S. The 'ding': amnestic states in football trauma. Neurology 1973 Feb;23(2):196-7.

137. Yarnell PR, Lynch S. Retrograde memory immediately after concussion. Lancet 1970 Apr 25;1(7652):863-4.

138. Oppenheimer DR. Microscopic lesions in the brain following head injury. J Neurol Neurosurg Psychiatry 1968 Aug;31(4):299-306.

139. Letter: Brain damage in sport. Lancet 1976 Mar 13;1(7959):585.

140. Harvey PK, Davis JN. Traumatic encephalopathy in a young boxer. Lancet 1974 Oct 19;2(7886):928-9.

141. Kaplan HA, Browder J. Observations on the clinical and brain wave patterns of professional boxers. J Am Med Assoc 1954 Nov 20;156(12):1138-44.

142. McCown IA. Protecting the boxer. J Am Med Assoc 1959 Mar 28;169(13):1409-13.

143. McCown IA. Boxing injuries. American Journal of Surgery 1959 September 1959;98:509-16.

144. Gonzales TA. Fatal injuries in competitive sports. J Am Med Assoc 1951 Aug 18;146(16):1506-11.

145. Parker HL. Traumatic Encephalopathy ('Punch Drunk') of Professional Pugilists. J Neurol Psychopathol 1934 Jul;15(57):20-8.

146. Winterstein CE. Head injuries attributable to boxing. The Lancet 1937 September 18, 1937;2:719-20.

147. Riffenburgh B, Barron B. The Official NFL encyclopedia. New York: New American Library; 1986.

148. California State Military Museum. Admiral Joseph Mason "Bull" Reeves, USN. 2012 [updated 2012; cited June 21, 2012]; Available from: http://www.militarymuseum.org/Reeves.html.

149. Daneshvar DH, Baugh CM, Nowinski CJ, McKee AC, Stern RA, Cantu RC. Helmets and mouth guards: the role of personal equipment in preventing sport-related concussions. Clin Sports Med Jan;30(1):145-63, x.

150. Viano DC, Pellman EJ, Withnall C, Shewchenko N. Concussion in professional football: performance of newer helmets in reconstructed game impacts--Part 13. Neurosurgery 2006 Sep;59(3):591-606; discussion 591-606.

151. Collins M, Lovell MR, Iverson GL, Ide T, Maroon J. Examining concussion rates and return to play in high school football players wearing newer helmet technology: a three-year prospective cohort study. Neurosurgery 2006 Feb;58(2):275-86; discussion -86.

152. McIntosh AS, McCrory P. Preventing head and neck injury. Br J Sports Med 2005 Jun;39(6):314-8.

153. Tagliabue P. Tackling concussions in sports. Neurosurgery 2003 Oct;53(4):796.

154. Pellman EJ, Viano DC, Tucker AM, Casson IR, Waeckerle JF. Concussion in professional football: reconstruction of game impacts and injuries. Neurosurgery 2003 Oct;53(4):799-812; discussion -4.

155. Pellman EJ, Viano DC. Concussion in professional football: summary of the research conducted by the National Football League's Committee on Mild Traumatic Brain Injury. Neurosurg Focus 2006;21(4):E12.

156. Pellman EJ, Viano DC, Tucker AM, Casson IR. Concussion in professional football: location and direction of helmet

impacts-Part 2. Neurosurgery 2003 Dec;53(6):1328-40; discussion 40-1.

157. Pellman EJ, Powell JW, Viano DC, Casson IR, Tucker AM, Feuer H, et al. Concussion in professional football: epidemiological features of game injuries and review of the literature--part 3. Neurosurgery 2004 Jan;54(1):81-94; discussion -6.

158. Pellman EJ, Viano DC, Casson IR, Tucker AM, Waeckerle JF, Powell JW, et al. Concussion in professional football: repeat injuries--part 4. Neurosurgery 2004 Oct;55(4):860-73; discussion 73-6.

159. Pellman EJ, Viano DC, Casson IR, Arfken C, Powell J. Concussion in professional football: injuries involving 7 or more days out--Part 5. Neurosurgery 2004 Nov;55(5):1100-19.

160. Pellman EJ, Lovell MR, Viano DC, Casson IR, Tucker AM. Concussion in professional football: neuropsychological testing--part 6. Neurosurgery 2004 Dec;55(6):1290-303; discussion 303-5.

161. Pellman EJ, Viano DC, Casson IR, Arfken C, Feuer H. Concussion in professional football: players returning to the same game--part 7. Neurosurgery 2005;56(1):79-90; discussion -2.

162. Viano DC, Pellman EJ. Concussion in professional football: biomechanics of the striking player--part 8. Neurosurgery 2005 Feb;56(2):266-80; discussion -80.

163. Pellman EJ, Lovell MR, Viano DC, Casson IR. Concussion in professional football: recovery of NFL and high school athletes assessed by computerized neuropsychological testing-Part 12. Neurosurgery 2006 Feb;58(2):263-74; discussion -74.

164. Viano DC, Casson IR, Pellman EJ, Bir CA, Zhang L, Sherman DC, et al. Concussion in professional football: comparison with boxing head impacts--part 10. Neurosurgery 2005 Dec;57(6):1154-72; discussion -72.

165. Viano DC, Casson IR, Pellman EJ, Zhang L, King AI, Yang

KH. Concussion in professional football: brain responses by finite element analysis: part 9. Neurosurgery 2005 Nov;57(5):891-916; discussion 891-916.

166. Viano DC, Casson IR, Pellman EJ. Concussion in professional football: biomechanics of the struck player--part 14. Neurosurgery 2007 Aug;61(2):313-27; discussion 27-8.

167. Pellman EJ, Viano DC, Withnall C, Shewchenko N, Bir CA, Halstead PD. Concussion in professional football: helmet testing to assess impact performance--part 11. Neurosurgery 2006 Jan;58(1):78-96; discussion 78-96.

168. Hamberger A, Viano DC, Saljo A, Bolouri H. Concussion in professional football: morphology of brain injuries in the NFL concussion model--part 16. Neurosurgery 2009 Jun;64(6):1174-82; discussion 82.

169. Viano DC, Hamberger A, Bolouri H, Saljo A. Concussion in professional football: animal model of brain injury--part 15. Neurosurgery 2009 Jun;64(6):1162-73; discussion 73.

170. Casson IR, Pellman EJ, Viano DC. Chronic traumatic encephalopathy in a National Football League player. Neurosurgery 2006 Nov;59(5):E1152.

171. Casson IR, Pellman EJ, Viano DC. Chronic traumatic encephalopathy in a National Football League player. Neurosurgery 2006 May;58(5):E1003; author reply E; discussion E.

172. Casson IR, Viano DC, Pellman EJ. Synopsis of the National Football League Player Health and Safety Meeting: Chicago, Illinois, June 19, 2007. Neurosurgery 2008 Jan;62(1):204-9; discussion 9-10.

173. Casson IR, Pellman EJ, Viano DC. Concussion in the national football league: an overview for neurologists. Neurol Clin 2008 Feb;26(1):217-41; x-xi.

174. Casson IR, Pellman EJ, Viano DC. Concussion in the National Football League: an overview for neurologists. Phys Med Rehabil Clin N Am 2009 Feb;20(1):195-214, x.

175. Casson IR, Pellman EJ, Viano DC. National football league experiences with return to play after concussion. Arch Neurol 2009 Mar;66(3):419-20.

176. Cassasa CB. Multiple traumatic cerebral hemorrhages. Proc New York Path Soc 1924 Jan. - May;24:101.

177. Royal College of Physicians of London. Committee on Boxing. Report on the medical aspects of boxing. London,: Royal College of Physicians of London; 1969.

178. Isherwood I, Mawdsley C, Ferguson FR. Pneumoencephalographic changes in boxers. Acta Radiol Diagn (Stockh) 1966;5:654-61.

179. Mawdsley C, Ferguson FR. Neurological Disease in Boxers. Lancet 1963 Oct 19;2(7312):799-801.

180. Spillane JD. Five boxers. Br Med J 1962 Nov 10;2(5314):1205-10.

181. Brennan TN, O'Connor PJ. Incidence of boxing injuries in the Royal Air Force in the United Kingdom 1953-66. Br J Ind Med 1968 Oct;25(4):326-9.

182. Guillain G, Sevileano E, Fandre M. [Not Available]. Bull Acad Natl Med 1948 Jun 8-15;132(21-22):394-406.

183. Guttmann E, Winterstein CE. Disturbances of consciousness after head injuries: observations on boxers. The British Journal of Psychiatry 1938;84(347-351).

184. Jokl E. The Medical Aspects of Boxing. Pretoria: J. L. Van Schaik, Ltd.; 1941.

185. Bergleiter R, Jokl E. [Brain injuries in boxing]. Zentralbl Neurochir 1956;16(1):28-44.

186. De Gispert Cruz I. Sobre la encefalopatía crónica de los boxeadores. Revista clínica espanõla 1943 November 30;11:270-3.

187. McAlpine D, Page F. Mid-brain syndrome in a professional boxer. Proc R Soc Med 1949 Oct;42(10):792.

188. Raevuori-Nallinmaa S. Brain injuries attributable to boxing. Acta Psychiatrica Scandinavica 1950 June 1950;25(S60):51-6.

189. Schwarz B. Chronische Schäden des Zentralnervensystems bei Boxern. . Dtsch Gesundh Wes 1953;8:845-7.

190. Lhermitte MJ. Discussion Remarks. Bulletin de l'Academie Nationale de Medecine 1948;132:405.

191. Taylor RB. Traumatic encephalopathy from boxing. Br Med J 1953 Jan 24;1(4803):200-1.

192. Geller W. [Paranoid psychosis due to boxing injuries]. Nervenarzt 1953 Feb 20;24(2):69-71.

193. Grahmann H, Ule G. [Diagnosis of chronic cerebral symptoms in boxers (dementia pugilistica & traumatic encephalopathy of boxers)]. Psychiatr Neurol (Basel) 1957 Sep-Oct;134(3-4):261-83.

194. Brandenburg W, Hallervorden J. [Dementia pugilistica with anatomical findings]. Virchows Arch 1954;325(6):680-709.

195. Soeder M, Arndt T. [Affective disorders and changes in the electroencephalogram of boxers]. Dtsch Med Wochenschr 1954 Nov 26;79(48):1792-5.

196. Wolowska J. [Encephalopathia pugilistica (boxer's disease)]. Neurol Neurochir Psychiatr Pol 1960 Nov-Dec;10:787-93.

197. Neubuerger KT, Sinton DW, Denst J. Cerebral atrophy associated with boxing. AMA Arch Neurol Psychiatry 1959 Apr;81(4):403-8.

198. Hese R, Sibielak J. [Pugilistic encephalopathy as a source of diagnostic errors]. Psychiatr Pol 1967 Jul-Aug;1(4):489-93.

199. Goralski H, Sypniewski J. [Boxing encephalopathy complicated by psychosis]. Neurol Neurochir Pol 1967 Sep-Oct;1(5):639-41.

200. Muller E. Diagnosis & evaluation of encephalopathy in boxers. Monatsschrift für Unfallheilkunde und Versicherungsmedizin 1958;61(4):117-23.

201. Henner K. Proæ. "musí být neurolog proti dnešní form" rohování? Casopis Lékaru Ceskych 1955;94(32):858-9.

202. La Cava G. [Not Available]. Brux Med 1949 Nov 6;29(45):3304-14.

203. La Cava G. [Not Available]. Brux Med 1949 Oct 30;29(44):3233; passim.

204. Pampus F, Grote W. [Electroencephalographic and clinical findings in boxers and their significance in the pathophysiology of traumatic brain disorders]. Arch Psychiatr Nervenkr Z Gesamte Neurol Psychiatr 1956;194(2):152-78.

205. Sercl M, Jaros O. [Mechanisms of closed head injuries in boxers and their sequelae]. Rozhl Chir 1962 Sep;41:597-600.

206. Sercl M, Jaros O. The mechanisms of cerebral concussion in boxing and their consequences. World Neurol 1962 May;3:351-8.

207. Temmes Y, Huhmar E. Electroencephalographic changes in boxers. Acta Psychiatr Neurol Scand 1952;27(1-2):175-80.

208. Carroll EJ. Punch Drunk. American Journal of the Medical Sciences 1936 May 1936;191(5):706-12.

209. Jokl E, Guttmann E. Neurologisch-psychiatrische Untersuchung an Boxern. Müch Med Wochenschr 1933;80:560-2.

210. Ravina A. [Results of electroencephalographic and cranial radiographic examination of boxers]. Presse Med 1955 Mar 19;63(21):419-20.

211. Ravina A. L'encephalite traumatique ou punch drunk. La Presse médicale 1937;45:1362-4.

212. Knoll W, Stille G, Herzog K. Boxschädigungen und ihre Verhütung. Arch Klin Chir 1938;191:36-42.

213. Benon R. [Neurological disorders among professional boxers]. Prog Med (Paris) 1950 Nov 24;78(22):583.

214. Graham JW. Professional boxing and the doctor. Br Med J 1955 Jan 22;1(4907):219-21.

215. Lobzin VS. [On closed injuries of the brain in boxers]. Zh Nevropatol Psikhiatr Im S S Korsakova 1960;60:542-6.

216. Boje O. Kroniske hjerneskader efter boksning. Ugeskrift For Laeger 1939 July 6, 1939;101:807-9.

217. Eiselt E. Effects of boxing on physical and mental health. Casopis Lékaru Ceskych 1948;87(26):766-9.

218. Rabadi MH, Jordan BD. The cumulative effect of repetitive concussion in sports. Clin J Sport Med 2001 Jul;11(3):194-8.

219. Saulle M, Greenwald BD. Chronic traumatic encephalopathy: a review. Rehabil Res Pract;2012:816069.

220. Daneshvar DH, Riley DO, Nowinski CJ, McKee AC, Stern RA, Cantu RC. Long-term consequences: effects on normal development profile after concussion. Phys Med Rehabil Clin N Am Nov;22(4):683-700, ix.

221. Gavett BE, Cantu RC, Shenton M, Lin AP, Nowinski CJ, McKee AC, et al. Clinical appraisal of chronic traumatic encephalopathy: current perspectives and future directions. Curr Opin Neurol Dec;24(6):525-31.

222. Gavett BE, Stern RA, McKee AC. Chronic traumatic encephalopathy: a potential late effect of sport-related concussive and subconcussive head trauma. Clin Sports Med Jan;30(1):179-88, xi.

223. Smodlaka VN. Medical aspects of heading the ball in soccer. Physician Sports Medicine 1984;12:127-31.

224. Tucker AM. Common soccer injuries. Diagnosis, treatment and rehabilitation. Sports Med 1997 Jan;23(1):21-32.

225. Matser JT, Kessels AG, Jordan BD, Lezak MD, Troost J. Chronic traumatic brain injury in professional soccer players. Neurology 1998 Sep;51(3):791-6.

226. Boden BP, Kirkendall DT, Garrett WE, Jr. Concussion incidence in elite college soccer players. Am J Sports Med 1998 Mar-Apr;26(2):238-41.

227. Tysvaer AT, Lochen EA. Soccer injuries to the brain. A neuropsychologic study of former soccer players. Am J Sports Med 1991 Jan-Feb;19(1):56-60.

228. Tysvaer AT. Head and neck injuries in soccer. Impact of minor trauma. Sports Med 1992 Sep;14(3):200-13.

229. Sortland O, Tysvaer AT. Brain damage in former association football players. An evaluation by cerebral computed tomography. Neuroradiology 1989;31(1):44-8.

230. Tysvaer AT, Storli OV. Soccer injuries to the brain. A neu-

rologic and electroencephalographic study of active football players. Am J Sports Med 1989 Jul-Aug;17(4):573-8.

231. Tysvaer AT, Storli OV, Bachen NI. Soccer injuries to the brain. A neurologic and electroencephalographic study of former players. Acta Neurol Scand 1989 Aug;80(2):151-6.

232. Tysvaer AT, Sortland O, Storli OV, Lochen EA. [Head and neck injuries among Norwegian soccer players. A neurological, electroencephalographic, radiologic and neuropsychological evaluation]. Tidsskr Nor Laegeforen 1992 Apr 10;112(10):1268-71.

233. Matser EJ, Kessels AG, Lezak MD, Jordan BD, Troost J. Neuropsychological impairment in amateur soccer players. JAMA 1999 Sep 8;282(10):971-3.

234. Powell JW, Barber-Foss KD. Traumatic brain injury in high school athletes. JAMA 1999 Sep 8;282(10):958-63.

235. Kelly JP, Rosenberg JH. The development of guidelines for the management of concussion in sports. J Head Trauma Rehabil 1998 Apr;13(2):53-65.

236. Collins MW, Grindel SH, Lovell MR, Dede DE, Moser DJ, Phalin BR, et al. Relationship between concussion and neuropsychological performance in college football players. JAMA 1999 Sep 8;282(10):964-70.

237. Kutner KC, Erlanger DM, Tsai J, Jordan B, Relkin NR. Lower cognitive performance of older football players possessing apolipoprotein E epsilon4. Neurosurgery 2000 Sep;47(3):651-7; discussion 7-8.

238. Jordan BD, Bailes JE. Concussion history and current neurological symptoms among retired professional football players. Neurology 2000;54(Suppl 3):A410-A1.

239. Honey CR. Brain injury in ice hockey. Clin J Sport Med 1998 Jan;8(1):43-6.

240. Jordan BD. Medical aspects of boxing. Boca Raton, Fla.: CRC Press; 1993.

241. Strich SJ. Diffuse degeneration of the cerebral white matter in severe dementia following head injury. Journal of Neurology,

Neurosurgery and Psychiatry 1956 August 1956;19(3):163 - 85.

242. Strich SJ. Shearing of the nerve fibers as a cause of brain damage due to head injury: a pathological study of twenty cases. . Lancet 1961 August 26, 1961;278(7200):443-98.

243. Pudenz RH, Shelden CH. The lucite calvarium; a method for direct observation of the brain; cranial trauma and brain movement. J Neurosurg 1946 Nov;3(6):487-505.

244. Martland HS, Beling CC. Traumatic cerebral hemorrhage. Archives of Neurology and Psychiatry 1929;22(5):1001-23.

245. Payne EE. Brains of boxers. Neurochirurgia (Stuttg) 1968 Sep;11(5):173-88.

246. Corsellis JA, Brierley JB. Observations on the pathology of insidious dementia following head injury. J Ment Sci 1959 Jul;105:714-20.

247. Constantinides J, Tissot R. Lésions neurofibrillaires d'Alzheimer généralisées sans plaques séniles. . Archives Suisses de Neurologie, Neurochirurgie et de Psychiatrie 1967;100:117-30.

248. Roberts GW. Immunocytochemistry of neurofibrillary tangles in dementia pugilistica and Alzheimer's disease: evidence for common genesis. Lancet 1988 Dec 24-31;2(8626-8627):1456-8.

249. Roberts GW, Allsop D, Bruton C. The occult aftermath of boxing. J Neurol Neurosurg Psychiatry 1990 May;53(5):373-8.

250. Rudelli R, Strom JO, Welch PT, Ambler MW. Posttraumatic premature Alzheimer's disease. Neuropathologic findings and pathogenetic considerations. Arch Neurol 1982 Sep;39(9):570-5.

251. Allsop D, Haga S, Bruton C, Ishii T, Roberts GW. Neurofibrillary tangles in some cases of dementia pugilistica share antigens with amyloid beta-protein of Alzheimer's disease. Am J Pathol 1990 Feb;136(2):255-60.

252. Tokuda T, Ikeda S, Yanagisawa N, Ihara Y, Glenner GG.

Re-examination of ex-boxers' brains using immunohisto-chemistry with antibodies to amyloid beta-protein and tau protein. Acta Neuropathol 1991;82(4):280-5.

253. Gabbita SP, Scheff SW, Menard RM, Roberts K, Fugaccia I, Zemlan FP. Cleaved-tau: a biomarker of neuronal damage after traumatic brain injury. J Neurotrauma 2005 Jan;22(1):83-94.

254. Smith DH, Chen XH, Nonaka M, Trojanowski JQ, Lee VM, Saatman KE, et al. Accumulation of amyloid beta and tau and the formation of neurofilament inclusions following diffuse brain injury in the pig. J Neuropathol Exp Neurol 1999 Sep;58(9):982-92.

255. Uryu K, Laurer H, McIntosh T, Pratico D, Martinez D, Leight S, et al. Repetitive mild brain trauma accelerates Abeta deposition, lipid peroxidation, and cognitive impairment in a transgenic mouse model of Alzheimer amyloidosis. J Neurosci 2002 Jan 15;22(2):446-54.

256. Yoshiyama Y, Uryu K, Higuchi M, Longhi L, Hoover R, Fujimoto S, et al. Enhanced neurofibrillary tangle formation, cerebral atrophy, and cognitive deficits induced by repetitive mild brain injury in a transgenic tauopathy mouse model. J Neurotrauma 2005 Oct;22(10):1134-41.

257. Smith DH, Chen XH, Pierce JE, Wolf JA, Trojanowski JQ, Graham DI, et al. Progressive atrophy and neuron death for one year following brain trauma in the rat. J Neurotrauma 1997 Oct;14(10):715-27.

258. Van Duijn CM, Clayton DG, Chandra V, Fratiglioni L, Graves AB, Heyman A, et al. Interaction between genetic and environmental risk factors for Alzheimer's disease: a reanalysis of case-control studies. EURODEM Risk Factors Research Group. Genet Epidemiol 1994;11(6):539-51.

259. Mortimer JA, van Duijn CM, Chandra V, Fratiglioni L, Graves AB, Heyman A, et al. Head trauma as a risk factor for Alzheimer's disease: a collaborative re-analysis of case-control studies. EURODEM Risk Factors Research Group. Int J Epidemiol 1991;20 Suppl 2:S28-35.

Table One

Omalu's constellation of CTE symptomatology, which was common to their CTE cohort

1. Long latent period between initial exposure to repeated blows to the head and manifestation of noticeable symptoms impairing activities of daily living
2. Progressive deterioration in socio-economic and cognitive functioning
   a. Loss of memory and memory disturbances
   b. Loss of previously acquired language and incoherence
   c. Loss of executive functioning
   d. Dismal business/investment performance
   e. Dismal money management
   f. Progressive deterioration in job performance and inability to maintain intellectually high performance jobs
   g. Deterioration in socio-economic status
   h. Bankruptcy
3. Paranoid ideations
   a. Social phobias
4. Exaggerated responses to life stressors
   a. Bouts of anger, worry and agitation over minor issues of daily living
5. Rampant fluctuations in mood [highs and lows; happy and sullen]
6. Breakdown of intimate and family relationships
   a. Spousal separation and divorces
7. Insomnia
8. Hyperactivity, restlessness, high energy level, high performance drive levels
   a. Poor attainment of set goals
   b. Dismal achievement levels in set tasks

9. Major depression
    a. Suicidal ideations and thoughts
    b. Suicide attempts/ completed suicides
10. Disinhibition and manifestation of poor judgment
    a. Criminal and violent tendencies and behavior
    b. Abuse of alcohol, prescription and illicit drugs
    c. Social indiscretions, sexual indiscretions, and sexual improprieties
    d. Increasing religiousity
11. Headaches, generalized body aches and pain

✒ ✒ ✒

Table Two

Osnato and Giliberti's Postconcussion Neurosis symptoms

Dizziness
Giddiness
Tinnitus
Visual Disturbances
  Blurred vision
  Subjective scotoma
  Optic atrophy
Headache
Pain in eyeballs
Nervous fears
Drowsiness
Hypersensitivities, especially to noises
Delirium
Restlessness
Depression
Disturbance of sleep
Sleeplessness at night
Irritability and moodiness
Emotionalism
Fatiguability
General weakness
Convulsion
Palpitation
Stuttering and stammering
Nausea
Vomiting

Table Three-A

Emerging gross and microscopic neuropathologic features of CTE

1. Brain may appear unremarkable or within normal limits for age on conventional Computerized Tomography [CT] Scanning and Magnetic Resonance Imaging [MRI] without cortical atrophy or ventriculomegaly

2. No xanthochromia of the dura mater or arachnoid mater, and no epidural or subdural membranes

3. No lobar cortical cavitatory contusional necrosis

4. No marked cortical lobar or subcortical ganglionic atrophy [Figure 1]

    a. Minimal to mild cortical atrophy of the frontal, parietal and temporal lobes may be present

    b. No hippocampal atrophy

    c. No cerebellar folial atrophy

    d. No brainstem atrophy

5. Normal pigmentation or minimal to mild hypopigmentation of the substantia nigra, locus ceruleus and/or dorsal raphe nucleus

6. No hydrocephalus ex-vacuo

7. Negligible, minimal to mild neocortical neuronal dropout

    a. No hippocampal sclerosis

8. Sparse to many subpial, subventricular and neuropil corpora amylaceae may be present

9. None to sparse multifocal perivascular infiltration of Virchow Robin spaces by few hemosiderin-laden histiocytes and lymphocytes, without vascular wall necrosis

10. Low grade, minimal to mild diffuse isomorphic fibrillary astrogliosis, subcortical white matter and centrum semiovale

11. Low grade, minimal to mild diffuse microglial activation and neuropil histiocytes, subcortical white matter and centrum semiovale

12. Low grade, minimal to mild rarefaction of the subcortical white matter and centrum semiovale

13. Sparse to frequent tau immunopositive neurofibrillary tangles and neuritic/neuropil threads, neocortex, subcortical ganglia and brainstem ganglia [Figure 2]

    a. Neurofibrillary tangles and neuropil threads in the cerebellar cortex, medial occipital cortex and calcarine cortex are extremely rare

    b. There may be neurofibrillary tangles in the neocortex, while relatively sparing the hippocampus

    c. Neurofibrillary tangles may assume different configurations: flame shaped, band shaped, small globose and large globose

    d. Ghost tangles may be present as well as tau immunopositive neuritic neuropil plaques

    e. Glial tau inclusions, astrocytic plaques, tufted and thorn astrocytes may be present but are frequently absent

    f. Neurofibrillary tangles and neuropil threads show random unpredictable differential topographic involvement of the neocortex showing a "skip-phenomenon", whereby different neocortical regions show no tangles or threads whatsoever, while other adjacent neocortical regions show sparse to frequent densities of tangles and threads in the same lobe.

    g. There may be larger numbers and densities of tangles and threads in the depths of the sulci and around blood vessels

    h. Sparse to frequent neurofibrillary tangles and neuropil threads with or without ghost tangles may be found in the subcortical ganglia and brainstem ganglia including the corpus striatum, thalamus, subthalamus, amygdala, nucleus accumbens, basal nucleus of Meynert, dorsal raphe nucleus, substantia nigra, locus ceruleus etc

    i. Involved subcortical and brainstem ganglia may show neuronal dropout

    j. Ubiquitin immunostains may highlight the neurofibrillary tangles and neuropil threads

14. Sparse to frequent diffuse amyloid plaques may be present in the neocortex, hippocampus, subcortical ganglia and brainstem nuclei [Figure 3]

a. None to sparse neuritic amyloid plaques may be present as well

b. Frequent neuritic amyloid plaques, like in AD, are more likely to be present in advanced or end stage CTE, especially in older patients

c. Cerebral amyloid angiopathy may or may not be present, but is frequently absent

15. There are no alpha-synuclein neuronal or glial inclusions; no Lewy bodies or Lewy neurites in the neocortex, subcortical ganglia and brainstem nuclei

a. The substantia nigra does not show Lewy bodies or Lewy neurites

16. Secondary Ubiquitin and TDP-43 proteinopathy may be present

✦ ✦ ✦

Table Three-B

Omalu-Bailes histomorphology subtypes of CTE

CTE SUB-TYPE	HISTOLOGIC FEATURES AND CRITERIA
0	Negative for CTE: NFTs and NTs absent in the cerebral cortex, subcortical nuclei/basal ganglia, brainstem and cerebellum
	No diffuse amyloid plaques in the cerebral cortex, subcortical nuclei/basal ganglia, brainstem or cerebellum
I	Sparse to frequent NFTs and NTs present in the cerebral cortex and brainstem, may be present in subcortical nuclei/basal ganglia
	No diffuse amyloid plaques in the cerebral cortex
	No NFTs and NTs in the cerebellum
2	Sparse to frequent NFTs and NTs present in the cerebral cortex and brainstem, may be present in subcortical nuclei/basal ganglia
	Sparse to frequent diffuse amyloid plaques present in the cerebral cortex
	No NFTs and NTs in the cerebellum
3	Moderate to frequent NFTs and NTs present in brainstem nuclei [brainstem predominant]
	None to sparse NFTs and NTs in cerebral cortex and subcortical nuclei/basal ganglia
	No NFTs and NTs in the cerebellum
	No diffuse amyloid plaques in the cerebral cortex

4   None to sparse [several] NFTs and NTs present in cerebral cortex, brainstem and subcortical nuclei/basal ganglia [incipient].

No NFTs and NTs in the cerebellum.

No diffuse amyloid plaques in the cerebral cortex

A   Moderate to frequent NFTs and NTs present in the hippocampus, diffuse amyloid plaques may or may not be present in the hippocampus

B   None to sparse NFTs and NTs in the hippocampus, diffuse amyloid plaques may or may not be present in the hippocampus

C   Sections of hippocampus unavailable for histological analysis

---

[NFT: Neurofibrillary Tangle; NT: Neuropil Thread]

This classification system is a two-tier system based on the presence or absence of NFTs, NTs and diffuse amyloid plaques in the cerebral cortex, subcortical nuclei/ basal ganglia, hippocampus and cerebellum; as well as the quantitative topographic distribution of NFTs and NTs in the cerebral cortex, subcortical nuclei/basal ganglia, hippocampus and cerebellum. The first tier classification has five subtypes represented by five Arabic numerals of 0, 1, 2, 3 and 4. The second tier classification has three subtypes represented by the first three capitalized letters of the English alphabet: A, B and C. This second tier classification applies to the presence or absence of NFTs and NTs, and to the quantitative distribution of NFTs and NTs in the hippocampus. Applying this classification scheme, each CTE case should be designated with either 0, 1, 2, 3 or 4 and A, B or C, connected with a hyphen. A negative CTE case is only represented as 0.

✐ ✐ ✐

Table Four

Syntactic maturation of CTE across the centuries: these are names CTE was recognized with across the centuries, listed in alphabetical order.

1. Cerebral neurasthenia
2. Chronic postconcussion syndrome
3. Chronic traumatic brain injury/chronic brain injury
4. Compensation hysteria
5. Concussion neurosis
6. Delayed traumatic apoplexy
7. Dementia pugilistica
8. Dementia traumatica
9. Encephalopathia traumatica
10. Litigation neurosis
11. Postconcussion neurosis
12. Postconcussion syndrome
13. Post-traumatic concussion state
14. Post-traumatic dementia
15. Post-traumatic head syndrome
16. Post-traumatic parkinsonism
17. Post-traumatic psychoneurosis
18. Post-traumatic stress disorder
19. Punch drunk/ punch drunk state
20. Terror neurosis
21. Traumatic constitution
22. Traumatic encephalitis
23. Traumatic encephalopathy
24. Traumatic encephalopathy of boxers
25. Traumatic hysterias
26. Traumatic insanity
27. Traumatic neurosis
28. Traumatic psychosis

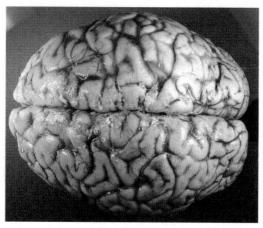

Figure 1a:
Gross photograph of Mike Webster's brain showing the dorsal surfaces of the cerebral hemispheres without any significant gross pathologic changes. Mike Webster was the very first confirmed CTE case in an American football player. Permission was obtained from the family and next-of-kin to publish these images.

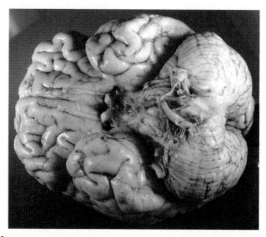

Figure 1b:
Gross photograph of Mike Webster's brain showing the basal surfaces of the brain without any significant gross pathologic changes.

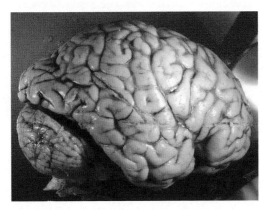

Figure 1c:
Gross photograph of Mike Webster's brain showing the right lateral surfaces of the brain without any significant gross pathologic changes.

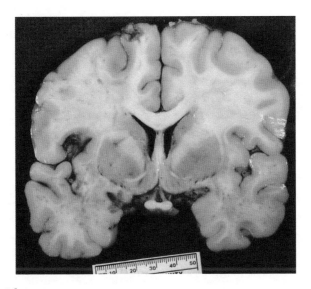

Figure 1d:
Gross photograph of Mike Webster's brain showing a coronal section of the cerebral hemispheres at the level of the anterior commissure showing no significant pathologic changes especially the absence of cortical or subcortical atrophy that would be seen in a brain with AD.

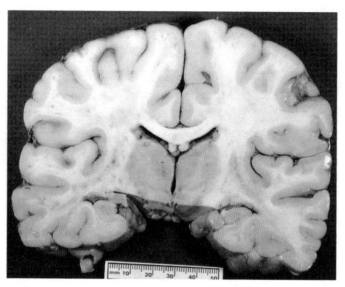

Figure 1e:
Gross photograph of Mike Webster's brain showing a coronal section of the cerebral hemispheres at the level of the cornu ammonis showing no significant pathologic changes especially the absence of hippocampal atrophy that would be seen in a brain with AD.

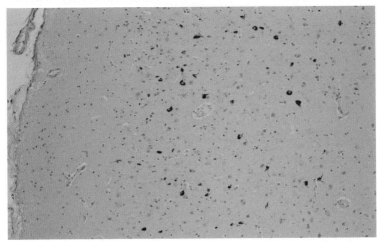

Figure 2a:
Photomicrograph of a tau-immunostained section of the neocortex from the brain of a retired NFL player with CTE showing frequent neurofibrillary tangles [x100 magnification]

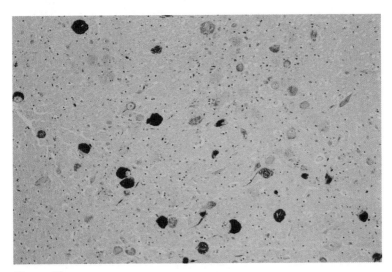

Figure 2b:
Photomicrograph of tau-immunostained section of a pigmented brainstem nucleus from the brain of a retired NFL player with CTE showing neuronal loss, frequent neurofibrillary tangles and neuropil threads, accompanied by scattered ghost tangles [x200 magnification]

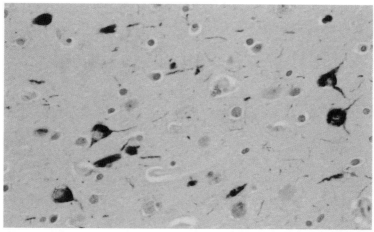

Figure 2c:
Photomicrograph of tau-immunostained section of the neocortex from the brain of a retired NFL player with CTE showing neurofibrillary tangles and neuropil threads [x400 magnification]

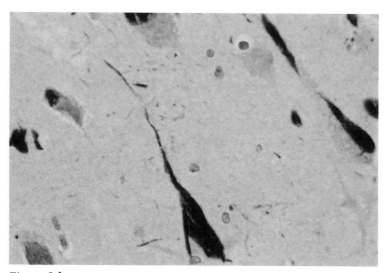

Figure 2d:
Photomicrograph of tau-immunostained section of the hippocampus from the brain of a retired NFL player with CTE showing neurofibrillary tangles and neuropil threads [x600 magnification]

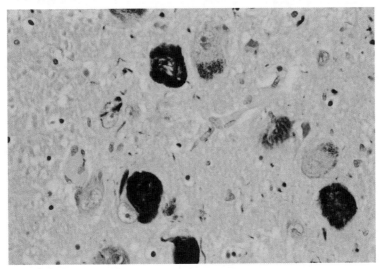

Figure 2e:
Photomicrograph of tau-immunostained section of the locus ceruleus from the brain of a retired NFL player with CTE showing globose and ghost neurofibrillary tangles and neuropil threads [x600 magnification]

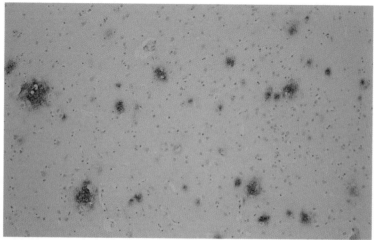

Figure 3a:
Photomicrograph of the BetaA4 amyloid immunostained section of the neocortex of Mike Webster's brain showing diffuse amyloid plaques [x100 magnification]

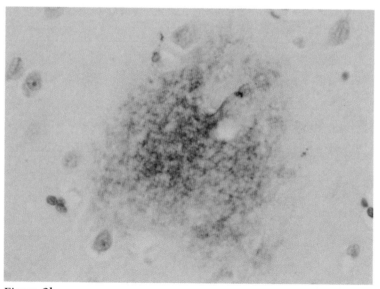

Figure 3b:
Photomicrograph of one of the diffuse amyloid plaques in the betaA4 immunostained section of Mike Webster's neocortex showing the absence of dystrophic neurites [x600 magnification]

Dr. Bennet Omalu was born to refugee parents in eastern Nigeria during the Biafra-Nigerian civil war. He survived the war and later attended medical school at the University of Nigeria, Enugu, Nigeria. He came to the United States in 1994 with a World Health Organization scholarship as a visiting scholar at the University of Washington, Seattle, Washington.

He completed residency training in anatomic pathology and clinical pathology at the College of Physicians and Surgeons of Columbia University, at Harlem Hospital Center, New York, New York. He completed fellowship training in forensic pathology at the Allegheny County Medical Examiner's Office, Pennsylvania, under Dr. Cyril Wecht. He completed fellowship training in neuropathology at the University of Pittsburgh, Pittsburgh, Pennsylvania. He completed a Masters in Public Health [MPH] program at the University of Pittsburgh, and a Masters in Business Administration [MBA] program at the Carnegie Mellon University, Pittsburgh, Pennsylvania.

Dr. Omalu is board certified in four specialties of medicine: anatomic pathology, clinical pathology, forensic pathology and neuropathology. He holds MPH and MBA degrees and is a certified physician executive [CPE]. He also holds a board certification in medical management awarded by the American College of Physician Executives. Dr. Omalu has been retained as an expert witness in forensic pathology, neuropathology and forensic science in thousands of cases in federal, state and county courts across the United States in both civil and criminal cases.

Dr. Omalu identified and described Chronic Traumatic Encephalopathy [CTE] in American football players beginning in 2002 when he performed an autopsy on Mike Webster. Between 2002 and 2007, Dr. Omalu identified the very first five cases of CTE in football players, and identified the very first case of CTE in a professional American wrestler in 2007 when he examined the brain of Chris Benoit. He also identified the first and second cases of CTE in war veterans when he examined the brains of a retired Vietnam war veteran, and a retired Iraq war veteran in 2007 and 2010 respectively.

Dr. Omalu published his first book *Play Hard, Die Young: Football Dementia, Depression and Death* in 2008. He lives in Lodi, California with his wife Prema Mutiso and their two children, Ashly and Mark.

Made in the USA
Lexington, KY
04 September 2015